ELECTROCARDIOGRAPHY FOR
THE ANAESTHETIST

ELECTROCARDIOGRAPHY
FOR THE
ANAESTHETIST

W. N. ROLLASON

M.B. M.R.C.S. D.A. F.F.A.R.C.S.

Regional Director of Anaesthetics
The Royal Infirmary, Aberdeen
Clinical Senior Lecturer in Anaesthetics
University of Aberdeen

WITH A FOREWORD BY

WILLIAM W. MUSHIN

M.A. M.B. B.S. F.F.A.R.C.S.
(HON.)F.F.A.R.A.C.S. F.F.A.R.C.S.I. F.F.A.(S.A.)

Professor of Anaesthetics
Welsh National School of Medicine

BLACKWELL
SCIENTIFIC PUBLICATIONS
OXFORD

TO MY WIFE

The good provider of that inestimable thing
a happy and a tranquil home

FIRST PUBLISHED 1964

Printed in Great Britain by

ADLARD & SON LTD, THE BARTHOLOMEW PRESS, DORKING

and bound by

THE KEMP HALL BINDERY, OXFORD

CONTENTS

v

FOREWORD

If the anaesthetist is to take notice of physiological changes in his patient and to relate his activities to them in a reasonable and flexible manner, he must receive continuous, reliable and quantitative information about these changes. The scientific instrument industry has been sensitive to this need and has responded quickly. There are now available highly developed devices for monitoring the main physiological systems of the body.

The problem facing the anaesthetist is interpretation. The barriers which have grown up round each field of medical knowledge often effectively prevent even basic information and terminology flowing readily from one field to another. It is essential and pressing that these barriers be broken down if the full benefit of the great advances in medical science be available to all who need them.

Electrocardiography is an example of this problem. The display and the recording of the electrical changes within the heart and their interpretation in terms of function and disease, is now widely practised and elaborate instruments to this end are readily available. Interested physicians all over the world devote their lives to a study of this matter and have developed great expertise and interpretive skill. The anaesthetist is realizing to an increasing extent the importance of electrocardiography as a source of information about the action of the heart, but he often lacks the ability to derive the fullest information from the electrocardiogram. As a result the accumulation of knowledge about the effects of anaesthesia on the heart is slow. But, just as the cardiologist will have to learn enough of anaesthesia to understand its relation to his field, and there are many obvious problems linking these two, so will the anaesthetist have to learn enough about cardiology and the electrocardiogram to predict, observe and minimize the harmful effects of his anaesthetics on the heart. This he must be able to do since the need arises in the operating theatre and other places where an expert colleague may not be available for advice.

Dr Rollason sets out to satisfy this need. His book is written by an anaesthetist for anaesthetists. The author does not aim to make his anaesthetist colleagues electrocardiographic experts, nor to displace or disdain the true expert in that field. He does, however, present a simple but accurate introduction to electrocardiography with particular reference to the electrical changes in the heart which occur in the special circumstances of modern anaesthesia. His own studies and contributions concerning electrocardiography during anaesthesia have been considerable. He speaks therefore not only as an anaesthetist, sensitive to the needs of his colleagues, but as one with some claim to expert knowledge of electrocardiography and its interpretation in anaesthesia.

His book will undoubtedly encourage more anaesthetists to use modern physiological monitoring instruments and to learn how to interpret and make use of the information they provide. In time these instruments will be accepted by all as essential aids to safe anaesthesia. Electrocardiography is without question one of the important major examples. In adopting this view and practice, anaesthetists will, while not lessening the content of art, increase enormously that of science, in anaesthesia.

WILLIAM W. MUSHIN
M.A. M.B. B.S. F.F.A.R.C.S.
(HON.)F.F.A.R.A.C.S. F.F.A.R.C.S.I.F.F. A.(S.A.)
Professor of Anaesthetics,
Welsh National School of Medicine

PREFACE

During the past decade the ECG has established itself as an important ancillary aid to the anaesthetist not only during surgery and anaesthesia, under the peculiar conditions of the operating theatre, but also in the pre- and post-operative periods. This aid, however, is only of value if the anaesthetist is capable of interpreting the significance of the changes it portrays.

While there are a number of standard works on electrocardiography, both introductory and comprehensive, available for study, they do not present the subject from the point of view of the anaesthetist, and it is hoped that this small volume may help to remedy this defect. In presenting it an endeavour has been made to steer between the Scylla of over-simplification and inadequate presentation on the one hand, and the Charybdis of complexity and lack of clarity on the other. It is however in no way intended to supplant any of the existing works on the subject, but rather to complement them.

I wish to extend my sincere thanks and appreciation to Dr D. S. Short and Mr J. M. Hough, M.A. who reviewed the manuscript and offered many helpful suggestions, which have been incorporated. I am also grateful to Mr Hough for his assistance in writing chapter VI. My grateful thanks are also due to Mr W. Topp for all the reproductions, to my secretary Mrs A. H. Dickson for her unstinting help, and to Professor W. W. Mushin for his generous foreword.

W. N. ROLLASON

Aberdeen
September 1963

ACKNOWLEDGMENTS

I am grateful to the following authors and publishers for permission to reproduce the illustrations indicated:

Dr B. S. Lipman and Year Book Medical Publishers Inc., Chicago for figs. 1, 19, 28, 31, 35, 40, 41, 60, 63–66, 68, 69 (from *Clinical Unipolar Electrocardiography*, 4th edn); Dr G. E. Burch and Henry Kimpton, London for figs. 6, 26, 27, 55, 56, 57 (from *A Primer of Electrocardiography*); Dr L. Schamroth and Blackwell Scientific Publications, Oxford for fig. 10 (from *An Introduction to Electrocardiography*); Dr J. E. F. Riseman and The Macmillan Company, New York for figs. 12a, b, c; 18 (from P.O.R.S.T.); Professor Saul D. Larks and Charles C. Thomas, Springfield, Illinois for fig. 20 (from *Fetal Electrocardiography*); Dr S. R. Arbeit and F. A. Davis Company, Philadelphia for figs. 21, 24, 25, 32, 34, 36–39, 42, 44–52, 61 (from *Differential Diagnosis of the Electrocardiogram*); Dr W. D. Wylie and Lloyd-Luke Ltd, London for figs. 30, 43, 53, 81 (from *A Practice of Anaesthesia*); Professor C. A. Keele and Professor Eric Neil and Oxford Medical Publications for figs. 11, 13, 17 (from Samson Wright's *Applied Physiology*, 10th edn).

I would also like to express my thanks to:

Dr Milton Kissin and the Editor of the *American Heart Journal* for fig. 5; Dr K. Lupprian, Dr H. Churchill-Davidson and the editor of the *British Medical Journal* for fig. 62; Dr M. Johnstone and the editor of the *British Journal of Anaesthesia* for figs. 70, 71, 74, 75; Dr J. H. Cannard and the Editor of *Anesthesiology* for figs. 72, 83; Dr J. G. Mudd and the Editor of the *American Heart Journal* for fig. 76a, b; Dr C. F. Scurr

ACKNOWLEDGMENTS

and the Editor of the *Proceedings of the Royal Society of Medicine* for fig. 82; Dr B. Benzon and the Editor of *Anaes-thesia* for fig. 84; Dr J. L. Eisaman and the Editor of the *American Journal of Surgery* for fig. 91.

CHAPTER I

INTRODUCTION

The heart muscle is unique among the muscles of the body in that it possesses the quality of automatic rhythmic contractions. These contractions produce weak electrical currents which spread through the entire body as the latter behaves like a volume conductor. The existence of these currents has been known for over a century. As early as 1856, Kölliker and Müller placed a frog's nerve muscle preparation in contact with a beating heart and were able to demonstrate twitches of the frog's muscles with each contraction of the ventricle. That these currents were measurable was demonstrated by Waller in 1887. He experimented with the capillary electrometer and recorded the electromotive force from the precordium. But it was not until 1901 when Einthoven invented his string galvanometer that the current from the human heart beat was registered in an accurate quantitative manner (Einthoven 1903). It was not, however, until 1918 that the human ECG was studied during anaesthesia (Krumbhaar 1918; Heard & Strauss 1918).

It is known that the electric impulse in the normal heart originates in the sino-atrial node and travels through both atria to reach the atrioventricular node. The excitation wave then passes to the bundle of His proceeding along its right and left branches to the Purkinge fibres in the ventricles. Activation of the ventricular musculature takes place initially in the septum and subsequently in the free walls of both ventricles. It is primarily the electrical activity within the cardiac muscle which is recorded on the electrocardiogram. It does not record haemodynamic events, such as the efficiency or force of contraction of the myocardium. The major portion of the muscle mass consists of the free walls of the right ventricle, the left ventricle and the septum. Similarly, the major portion of the completed electrocardiogram consists of the electrical activity present in the septum and the two ventricles.

A cell is said to be polarized in the resting state, meaning that an equal number of ionic charges of opposite polarity (negative and positive) is present on both sides of the cell membrane. The positively charged ions (cations) are distributed on the outer surface and the negatively charged ions (anions) within (Curtis & Cole 1941).

Stimulation makes the cell membrane permeable to the flow of ions, so that a flow of current occurs. On stimulation, depolarization locally ensues, and this depolarized locus is propagated along the cell membrane, setting up a moving boundary of potential difference between the stimulated and the resting areas. At the head of the advancing locus of activity, where the depolarized muscle encounters the boundary of the resting polarized muscle, a series of dipoles appear (Ashman 1948). A dipole consists of a positive and a negative charge in close proximity to each other and of equal magnitude. Stimulation of the resting muscle thus produces an advancing wave of activity represented by a series of dipoles which are propagated along the cell membrane and form a moving boundary of potential difference and this phenomenon is recordable.

Such a potential difference must be present between two electrodes in order to record a deflection. If there is no difference in potential, as in a zone of completely active or completely inactive muscle, no electrocardiographic deflections will be recorded.

Each mechanical contraction is accompanied by two electrical processes, depolarization (activation) and repolarization (recovery). The advancing dipoles are so orientated during depolarization that the positive ion precedes the negative ion, i.e. the head is positive and the tail negative. When the muscle has been completely depolarized, it is referred to as apolarized. Repolarization then occurs and the outside of the membrane recovers its resting charge. During this process of repolarization the dipole is reversed, i.e. the head is negative and the tail positive. This is illustrated in Fig. 1.

The electrocardiogram is the graphic representation of the electrical forces produced by the heart. Einthoven correlated the contracting heart with the electrocardiographic waves it produced and demonstrated that the P wave was related to the atrial contraction,

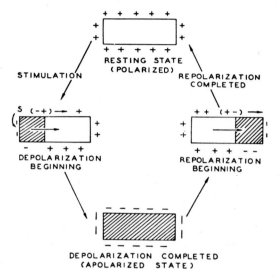

FIG. 1. Electrical activity associated with one contraction in a muscle fibre.

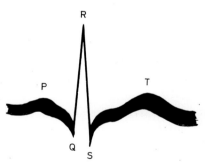

FIG. 2. Normal limb lead tracing.

whereas the QRS complex and the T wave were associated with the ventricular contraction. The waves produced by a normal cardiac contraction are shown in Fig. 2.

CHAPTER II

THE NORMAL ECG

From the point of view of electric currents, the heart consists of two complex systems of cells, one constituting the atria and the other the ventricles, so that electrocardiographically, each system may be considered separately. Each mechanical contraction, atrial and ventricular, is associated with two electrical processes, i.e. depolarization and repolarization, illustrated in Fig. 1. Depolarization of the ventricles is represented by the QRS complex and repolarization by the T wave. The ST segment represents the period when all parts of the ventricles are in the depolarized or apolarized state. Depolarization of the atria is represented by the P wave; repolarization also occurs although the electrical record is usually obscured by the QRS complex, so that the T wave of the atrium— the Ta wave—is not normally seen. The atrial T wave (unlike that of the ventricle) is normally negative, i.e. below the base line. The base line is termed 'iso-electric'. The U wave is a wave low in magnitude following the T wave and is of little practical significance.

The PR and PQ interval, measured from the beginning of the P wave to the onset of the R or Q wave, respectively, marks the time which an impulse leaving the sinus node takes to reach the ventricles. The PR interval is normally not less than 0·12 second and not over 0·2 second.

The QRS interval measured from the beginning of the Q wave to the end of the S wave, represents the process of depolarization of the ventricles. During this time the cardiac impulse travels first through the interventricular system and then through the free walls of the ventricles. It normally varies from 0·05 to 0·10 second. The normal intervals are illustrated in Fig. 3.

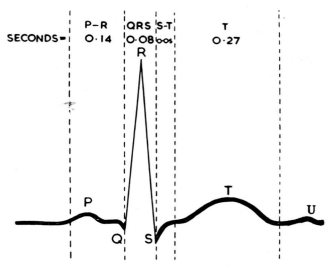

Fig. 3. Normal limb lead tracing illustrating the intervals.

The system is depolarized from the left to the right because a small branch of the left bundle of His is given off first. The subendo cardial regions of the ventricles are activated before the adjacent myocardial and subepicardial areas (Fig. 4).

The T wave represents repolarization of both ventricles. Hence one complete ventricular contraction (systole) is represented by the QT interval measured from the beginning of the Q wave to the end of the T wave. This interval varies with age, sex and cardiac rate. When the rate is rapid, the interval is short and vice versa,

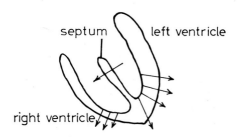

Fig. 4. Mechanism of ventricular depolarization.

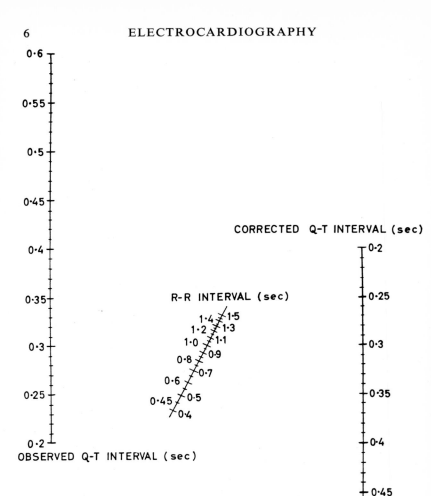

FIG. 5. Nomogram for rate correction of QT interval. Measure the observed QT interval and the RR interval. Mark these values in the respective columns of the chart (left and middle): connect these two points with a ruler and extend this line until it intersects the QTc column; this will be the QTc interval.

e.g. at cardiac rates of 60–70 it is in the region of 0·4 second. The QTc interval is the QT interval corrected for cardiac rate from the formula $QTc = QT\sqrt{c}$ where c is the cycle length, which is 1 second when the pulse rate is 60 per minute and QTc = QT. It can be calculated for other pulse rates by means of a slide rule when the actual QT interval and cycle length are known. The QTc interval may also be obtained from the nomogram which is illustrated in Fig. 5.

Ventricular diastole extends from the end of the T wave to the beginning of the next Q wave.

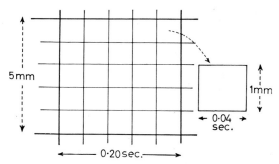

Fig. 6. Time markings and voltage lines of the electrocardiogram.

Horizontal and vertical lines appear on all electrocardiograms. The vertical lines represent time and are divided into larger and smaller squares. A large square indicates 0·2 second and a small square 0·04 second. The horizontal lines represent voltage, 1 mm being equal to 0·1 mV, when the current is correctly standardized (Fig. 6).

To calculate the rate, the number of QRS complexes (for ventricular rate) or P waves (for atrial rate) occurring in a certain period of time are counted, e.g. the number of QRS complexes occurring in 3 seconds (15 large squares) is counted and multiplied by 20 to calculate the ventricular rate per minute. Most recording graphs have every fifteenth square marked by a vertical line at the upper border of the strip. Alternatively, the rule illustrated in Fig. 7 may

—HEART RATE PER MINUTE—

FIG. 7. The arrow should be placed on a heart complex (P or QRS) and the rate is obtained when the scale intersects the same portion of a complex two cycles removed. (Applicable for regular rhythm only).

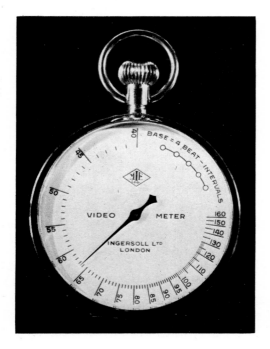

FIG. 8. The videometer. This is wound in an anticlockwise direction. By depressing the single control it will start, stop or zero the pointer sequentially.

be used. When the tracings are displayed on an ECG monitor, a videometer may be employed. This is hand operated and will record a reading of heart rate within a range of 40 to 160 per minute. It is illustrated in Fig. 8 and its method of use in Fig. 9.

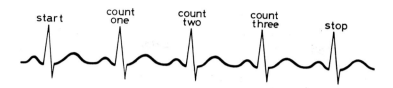

Fig. 9. Assuming the operator is viewing an ECG tracing the control having been wound and the pointer zeroed, is pressed to start at the first observed tracing and the next three tracings counted. At the fourth tracing the control is pressed to stop as shown. The pointer will then be observed at the figure representing the rate per minute.

THE ECG LEADS

STANDARD LEADS

These were introduced by Einthoven at the beginning of the century and have been adopted as the standard leads throughout the world.

Two electrodes placed over different areas of the heart and connected to the galvanometer will pick up the electrical currents resulting from the potential difference between them. For example, if under the first electrode a wave of 0·2 mV, and under the second electrode a wave of 0·6 mV occur over the same period of time, then the two electrodes will record the difference between them, i.e. a wave of 0·4 mV. A bipolar lead, therefore, records all electrical events between the two terminals by revealing the changes of one electrode over and above the changes affecting the other. The final tracing of the ECG is thus a composite recording of both electrodes.

In standard lead I the terminals are placed on the right and left arms (RA and LA). In lead II, the terminals are placed on the right arm and left leg (RA and LF–F = foot) and in lead III the terminals are placed on the left arm and the left leg (LA and LF).

In the standard leads the P wave should be upright in lead I and usually in lead II, but may be inverted in lead III. It should not be more than 2·0 mm in height or 0·1 second in duration.

Q must be small in leads I and II, but may be deep in lead III.

R should be at least 5 mm high in any one of the three tracings and no higher than 15 mm in any lead.

The ST interval should not be displaced more than 1 mm above or below the isoelectric line.

The T wave should be upright in lead I and II, or possibly diphasic in II, but may be inverted in lead III. It should be at least 2 mm high in one of these leads.

UNIPOLAR LEADS (V LEADS)

Here again, two electrodes are employed, but because one is inactive (the neutral or indifferent electrode) and has no electrical changes occurring in its vicinity, the electrocardiographic tracing mirrors potential alterations taking place only in the vicinity of the other, the active, or exploring, electrode.

To appreciate how one electrode has a zero potential the heart may be considered to be in the centre of an equilateral triangle, the apices of which are the right arm, left arm and left leg leads (Fig. 10). According to Einthoven, the algebraic sum of the potentials of these three leads is at any instant equal to zero. Thus if these three leads are connected to a central terminal, the potential of this terminal will be zero (Fig. 10). In practice there is also a high resistance inserted in this central terminal.

If this central terminal which constitutes the inactive, neutral, or indifferent electrode is connected to one lead of a galvanometer, that lead will always have a potential value of zero. The electrode connected to the other lead of the galvanometer will then record the true potential at any given point. This electrode constitutes the active or exploring electrode. It is also referred to as the V or 'voltage' lead.

Two types of unipolar leads are employed (a) limb leads and (b) precordial leads.

(a) *Limb leads*. The potential value in the right arm may be obtained by connecting the exploring electrode to the right arm and the indifferent electrode to the other terminal of the galvanometer. This lead is termed VR. A similar technique is employed for obtaining the left arm and left leg extremity leads VL and VF respectively. The unipolar limb lead tracings are illustrated in Fig. 11.

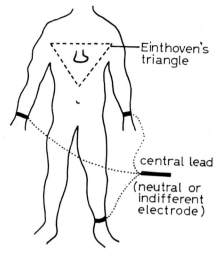

FIG. 10. Einthoven's triangle and the central terminal.

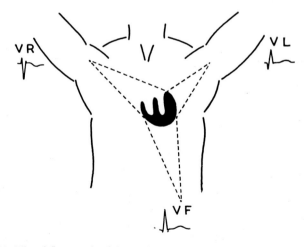

FIG. 11. The right arm lead faces the cavity of the ventricle, the left leg lead faces the inferior surface of the heart; this may be formed by the right or left ventricle or both, depending on the position of the heart. The left arm lead may face the cavity of the ventricles or the outside of the left ventricle, depending on the position of the heart. (Diagram by Dr D. S. Short.)

As the potential obtained by the exploring exlectrode of these leads is of low voltage the latter is usally augmented (A) by omitting the connection of the neutral terminal to the limb which is being tested. Thus the augmented unipolar limb leads are referred to as AVR, AVL and AVF respectively.

(b) *Precordial leads*. The second type of unipolar lead is a precordial lead and utilizes an exploring electrode to record the electrical potential of the right ventricle, septum and left ventricle.The unipolar chest leads are designated by the single capital letter 'V', followed by a subscript numeral which represents the location of the electrode on the precordium. Six chest positions are routinely used (V1–6):

V1: 4th intercostal space to right of sternum.
V2: ,,   ,,   ,, ,, left ,,   ,,
V3: Midway between left sternal border and mid-clavicular line on a line joining positions 2 and 4.
V4: 5th intercostal space in mid-clavicular line.
V5: ,,   ,,   ,, ,, left anterior axillary line.
V6: ,,   ,,   ,, ,, ,, mid-axillary line.

The position of the chest leads are illustrated in Fig. 12a, b and c.

C LEADS

In this type of lead which like the standard lead is bipolar in character the exploring C (chest) electrode is coupled with a relatively indifferent electrode placed either on the right arm (CR), left arm (CL), or left leg (CF). C leads are V-leads minus the potentials in VR, VL and VF. As VR potentials are negative, their subtraction from V in CR records make all deflections more positive. This may be useful in demonstrating P waves of low voltage which may not be obvious in other leads; alternatively the P wave can be detected in an oesophageal lead, but this is not routinely employed. The CL and CF leads are now rarely used.

The normal standard, augmented and precordial leads are illustrated in Fig. 13 and the C leads are compared with the standard leads in Fig. 14.

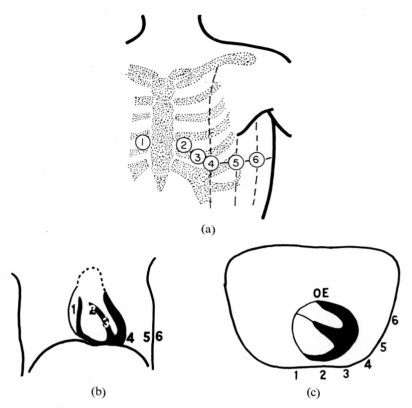

(a)

(b)   (c)

FIG. 12. (a) Position of the exploring electrodes on the precordium.
(b) The cardiac structures visualized by the precordial exploring
electrodes.
(c) The cardiac structure visualized by both the precordial electrodes
and the oesophageal electrode (OE).

ELECTRICAL ACTIVITY OF THE VENTRICLES

By convention, a wave is inscribed above the isoelectric line, i.e.
positive when depolarization travels towards the exploring electrode from a remote area. It follows, therefore, that when an exploring electrode is placed over the right ventricle, it will receive
an initial positive electrical impulse from septal depolarization (1),
and a delayed negative impulse from left ventricular wall depolar-

3

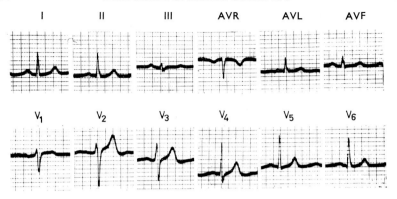

FIG. 13. Normal 12 lead ECG.

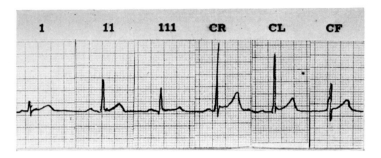

FIG. 14. Standard and C leads.

ization (2). The tracing of the right ventricular wall therefore is a RS complex as seen in Fig. 15.

Similarly, a left ventricular wall complex is composed of an initial negative septal current, and a later positive lateral wall current or a QR complex (Fig. 16).

Because of the relationship of the cardiac septum to the chest wall, the Q wave is not normally deep (1·5 mm or less). Therefore, as the exploring electrode is moved from the right ventricle over the chest to the left, the tracing evolves from the RS wave toward the QR complex. This progression from right to left is character-ized by a gradual elevation of the R as the S becomes more shallow, until R about equals the S in magnitude as the electrode overlies the septum. This is called the transitional zone. Farther left, S becomes very small and in many tracings S will disappear and leave the QR complex in position V6, thus completing the evolution. These changes are illustrated in Fig. 17.

The smoothness of progression of the QRS complex is influenced by a third factor besides the septal and lateral wall currents. This

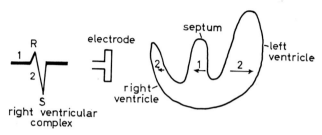

FIG. 15. The right ventricular complex.
(In the normal heart the larger left ventricular forces counteract and in effect nullify the smaller forces of the right ventricle so that septal depolarization (1) and left ventricular depolarization (2) need only be considered.)

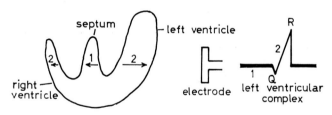

FIG. 16. The left ventricular complex.

is the positive tendency of endo-epicardial depolarization taking place directly under the electrode. R in V 5 and 6 may not be quite as tall, because the heart recedes from the chest wall as the axilla is approached. Moreover, reduction in voltage of R in V 1–3 may be due in women to resistance of breast tissue. If R suddenly becomes small in any position as observation is made from right to left, disease is probably present.

The T wave in V 1 and 2 may be negative, but should be unalterably upright beyond position 2 in adults.

The ST interval should normally vary between isoelectric and plus 2 mm. (Contrast with 1 mm in the standard leads.) The ST segment should never be negative or higher than 2 mm.

Of less importance is the fact that R should not exceed 25 mm and that P, like T, may be negative in V 1 and 2.

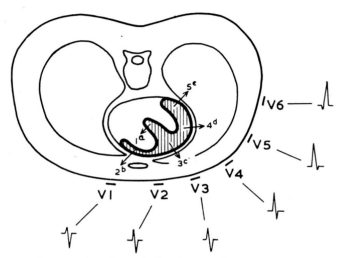

FIG. 17. Cross section through the chest to show thep recordial leads and their relation to the heart; a, b, c, d and e show the order in which the electrical impulse spreads through the ventricle. Note the alteration in the configuration of the QRS complex between V1 and V6. (Diagram by Dr D. S. Short.)

CLOCKWISE AND COUNTER-CLOCKWISE ROTATION OF THE HEART

The longitudinal axis of the heart runs obliquely from apex to the base of the heart. Rotation round this axis is conventionally viewed from below the heart looking towards the apex. This rotation is clockwise or counter-clockwise and either position can be normal.

In clockwise rotation the right ventricle assumes an anterior position and the precordial leads will record right ventricular or RS complexes in the V4–6 positions.

In counter-clockwise rotation the left ventricle will rotate anteriorly so that now both right and left ventricles assume an anterior position and QR complexes may be seen in the V3–6 positions.

ELECTRICAL POSITION OF THE HEART

Variations in the anatomical position of the heart are reflected electrically by the ECG.

In the neutral position, the anterior cardiac surface is largely right ventricle, and the apex and left border are composed of left ventricular wall. When the heart becomes horizontal it rotates round its antero-posterior axis which runs through the centre of the septum from the anterior to the posterior surface so that the left ventricle faces the left shoulder, and the right ventricle faces the left foot. Therefore, AVL (left arm) resembles the QR or left ventricular complex and AVF (left foot), the RS or right ventricular complex.

When the heart becomes vertical, the opposite event occurs and AVL tends to the RS right ventricular complex and AVF toward a QR left ventricular complex. In determining the position of the heart it is advisable to base the findings only on the location of the QR complex. When the heart occupies a neutral or intermediate position, the complexes of AVL and AVF tend to be the same, either the RS or the QR pattern. The positions of the heart and associated axis changes (see Chapter III) are illustrated diagrammatically in Fig. 18.

The AVR complex rarely enters the field of interpretation of the electrical position of the heart. Normally the AVR active electrode always faces some aspect of the cavity of the heart. The septal current runs mostly or entirely perpendicular to the electrode and causes either a small or no deflection at all. The lateral ventricular wall, however, produces a negative complex because depolarization travels away from the electrode which faces the cavity. In short, AVR normally is negative.

As the electrode is moved more posteriorly, it faces not only part of the ventricular orifices or cavity, but also the posterior wall itself. The electrode is still perpendicular to the septum and no septal current occurs and the cavity still produces a negative wave. The posterior wall current, however, just over the electrode proceeds as usual from endocardium to epicardium and therefore towards this posterior electrode. A late positive wave results. The complex for the posterior wall of the heart is thus a deep QR. This deep cavity Q must not be confused with the shallow septal Q.

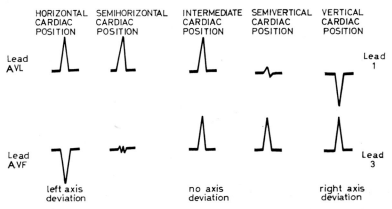

FIG. 18. The five patterns in the unipolar limb leads which indicate the cardiac position compared with the three patterns in the standard leads indicating axis deviation.

NORMAL VARIANTS OF THE ADULT PATTERN

Up to the time of birth, the foetal heart has had to provide a circulation through both the body tissues and the placental mass. The additional load is, by virtue of the patent ductus, shared between the right and left ventricles. As a result, at birth the development of the two ventricles is approximately equal, i.e. their wall thickness is similar. As a consequence, the ECG pattern simulates that of right ventricular hypertrophy in the adult (see Chapter III). This is associated with tall R waves and inverted T waves in the right precordial leads and is illustrated in Fig. 19.

In children, the tall R waves in the right precordial leads usually disappear after the age of five, but inverted T waves in the precordial leads frequently persist into the second decade.

In negroes this 'juvenile pattern' of T wave inversion in the precordial leads may persist into the third decade of life.

In older children, as in adults, an inverted T wave is common in V1. In the precordial leads, a negative T wave with a positive T wave in a position to the right of it is considered abnormal, so for a proper interpretation of the juvenile ECG leads V1–6 should be examined.

The child's heart is usually in the vertical position and only rarely in the horizontal position.

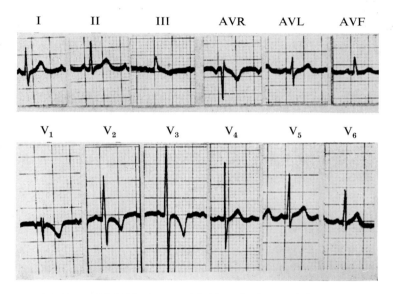

FIG. 19. Normal ECG in boy aged 2. Note the inverted T waves in V1, V2 and V3 which are normal at this age.

THE FOETAL ECG

Much work has been done on foetal electrocardiography in the United States (Larks 1961), but so far it has not been regarded as a practical proposition in Great Britain, certainly during labour when interference is gross due to the superimposition of artefacts from movement and skin currents. The maternal ECG is also

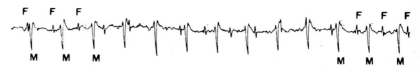

Fig. 20. The foetal complexes (F) can be distinguished from the
maternal complexes (M).

present in the tracing but can usually be distinguished by a difference in amplitude and frequency. The foetal ECG is illustrated in
Fig. 20. More recently, however, Kendall *et al* (1962) have evolved
a system of radio-electrocardiography which is almost completely
free from electrical interference, and in future it should be possible
to provide accurate information about the condition of the foetus
in utero.

CHAPTER III

THE ABNORMAL ECG

Abnormal patterns may be associated with changes in the configuration of the P wave, QRS complex, ST segment and T wave, or by alteration in the PR, QRS and QT intervals. In addition, there may be disorders of cardiac rhythm. These abnormal patterns may be due to pathological states, but on occasion they may be due to artefact.

ALTERATIONS IN THE P WAVE

The P wave is tall and sharp, the height ranging from 2 to 5 mm in right atrial hypertrophy, e.g. in pulmonary stenosis, and is referred to as P pulmonale.

It is usually bifid and conspicuously widened, the duration being in the region of 0·12 second, in left atrial hypertrophy, e.g. in mitral stenosis, and is referred to as P mitrale. It is often best seen in standard lead II.

It is widened and the voltage is low in hypertensive or aortic valve disease.

In lead I it is inverted in dextrocardia. This is illustrated in Fig. 21.

It may be inverted in leads II and III in superior nodal (coronary sinus) rhythm.

It may be inverted in leads I, II and III in inferior nodal rhythm.

It may be rendered unrecognizable by muscular tremors, such as shivering, so that determination of the site of the pace maker becomes impossible. The configuration of the P wave frequently changes in height and direction when the pace maker shifts from

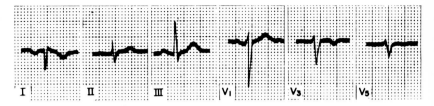

FIG. 21. Congenital Dextrocardia. Lead I is the mirror image of normal lead I; leads II and III are reversed and leads V3 and 5 resemble the right precordial leads.

the sinus node to varying portions of the atrium and the PR interval varies. This phenomenon is called Wandering pace maker and will be referred to again under ectopic rhythm.

ALTERATIONS MAINLY AFFECTING THE QRS COMPLEX

AXIS DEVIATION

In Fig. 22, the normal electrical cardiac axis is indicated by the arrow RA → LF, the length depending on the voltage. Its direction indicates an electrode link-up of right arm to left foot. This axis can be broken up into its horizontal or lead I (RA → LA) and vertical or lead III (LA → LF) vectors or components. Since a positive wave is inscribed when depolarization proceeds from

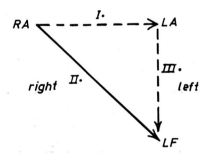

FIG. 22. The normal electrical cardiac axis.

RA to LF, then its two components, i.e. RA to LA to LF are similarly positive. Normal axis is seen in Fig. 13 (standard leads). When the electrical axis of a heart shows left axis deviation of marked degree, the horizontal axis points not only toward the left shoulder but to a landmark above it. Such left axis deviation is illustrated in Fig. 23.

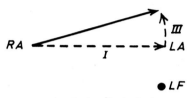

FIG. 23. Left axis deviation.

Lead I reveals positive depolarization from RA to LA, but lead III indicates a negative wave, in that depolarization travels from LA away from LF. Left axis deviation, therefore, manifests itself in a large R possibly with a small Q (left ventricular pattern) in lead I, and a negative complex or small R, and very deep S (right ventricular pattern) in lead III. This is illustrated in Fig. 24.

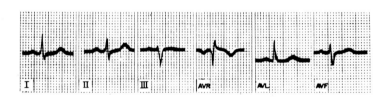

FIG. 24. Left axis deviation (leads I and III). Horizontal heart (leads AVL and AVF).

In marked right axis deviation, the electrical axis points to the right of the vertical, and therefore, the QRS complex in lead I is negative (from LA to RA) and that in lead III is positive (Fig. 25).

Negativity is produced by the S wave. If it were produced by the Q wave it would imply not axis deviation but infarction.

As leads I and III are the vectors of lead II, the waves in lead II are almost an addition of the other two leads.

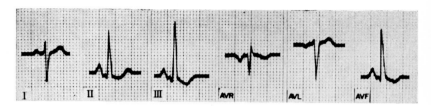

FIG. 25. Right axis deviation (leads I and III). Vertical heart (leads AVL and AVF).

Axis deviation may also be expressed in degrees (minus or plus, i.e. counter-clockwise or clockwise respectively), from the three o'clock axis (lead I line) of a triaxial system (Bayley 1943). Fig. 26 illustrates the three types of axis deviation for the QRS complex, i.e. (1) normal axis deviation when the axis is between 0 and +90°, (2) right axis deviation when the axis is more positive than 90° and (3) left axis deviation when the axis is more negative than 0°.

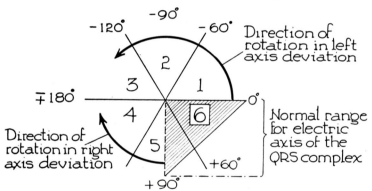

FIG. 26. The range of the normal axis of the QRS complex in degrees and the direction of rotation in left or right axis deviation.

Axis deviation may be obtained from a calculator (Rumball 1963) or from Dieuaide's chart (Fig. 27). It may also be calculated from the formula

$$\tan V = \frac{\dfrac{l_3}{l_1} + \frac{1}{2}}{0 \cdot 866} \, 0$$

where V is the direction of the electric axis in degrees, l_1 is the electric vector in mm for lead I and is the algebraic sum of the R and S peaks in this lead, and l_3 is similarly the electric vector for lead III.

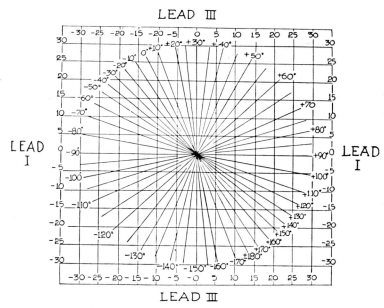

FIG. 27. Dieuaide's chart for finding electric axis. To determine the electric axis of the QRS complex: the algebraic sum of the positive and negative deflections of the QRS complex in lead I is plotted along the lead I line (ordinate) and the algebraic sum of the positive and negative deflections of the QRS complex in lead III is plotted along the lead III line (abscissa). Perpendicular lines are drawn to these points. The point of junction of these perpendiculars represents the tip of the arrowhead of a vector force of the QRS axis, the tail being at zero or centre of the graph. The angle can be determined by the angle lines of the graph nearest the vector formed.

The direction of the mean normal electrical axis varies considerably with the age of the subject. In the infant under 6 months of age, the axis is greatly to the right ($+130°$). Between the ages of one and five years, the axis moves to the left, the average for these ages inclusive being about $+52°$. The axis then returns to the right at puberty, the average axis being about +67°. It again returns to the left in the adult, averaging about +58°. These changes in position are due mainly to the changing position of the heart in the thorax, except in the case of the infant.

Left axis deviation is present in (1) 10 per cent of normal people who are usually hypersthenic subjects, (2) left ventricular hypertrophy and dilatation, (3) left bundle branch block, (4) cardiac displacement to the left, e.g. due to scoliosis, elevation of the diaphragm as a result of pregnancy, obesity or ascites. It is associated with such diseases as aortic stenosis or incompetence, hypertension, mitral incompetence, coarctation of the aorta, arterio-venous aneurysm, and ostium primum defect.

Right axis deviation is present in (1) the newborn (2) 10 per cent of normal children over the age of 8 years (3) right ventricular hypertrophy and dilatation (4) right bundle branch block and (5) cardiac displacement to the right. It is associated with such diseases as emphysema, mitral and pulmonary stenosis, and ostium secundum defect.

VOLTAGE CHANGES

An excessively high or low voltage of the QRS complex may be due to a standardization error and this should be checked. On the other hand it may be related to the thickness of the chest wall and to disease.

High voltage may be seen in patients with (1) a thin chest wall (2) ventricular hypertrophy and (3) hyperthyroidism.

Low voltage may be seen in patients with (1) a thick chest wall (2) a pericardial effusion, anasarca, myocarditis or myopathy (3) myxoedema and (4) carbon monoxide poisoning.

In order to distinguish between axis and voltage changes of the QRS complex, the simultaneous observation of at least two of the standard leads is necessary (Rollason & Hough 1957a).

LEFT VENTRICULAR HYPERTROPHY

This is classically seen in patients with hypertension and is associated with left axis deviation. The diagnostic electrocardiographic signs are:—

(1) The R wave is likely to exceed 15 mm in one of the standard leads because of the generation of excess voltage.

(2) The tall R wave is followed by an inverted T wave. When the myocardium is severely hypertrophied or 'strained' it has been conjectured that the wave of repolarization or T wave is so retarded in its progress through the affected myocardium that other areas set up their own wave of repolarization. Consequently, a reverse progression occurs which imparts to the tracing a negative T.

(3) There is a delay in the onset of the downstroke of the R wave (the intrinsicoid deflection) over the left ventricular leads. Almost all the voltage changes concerned with the R wave in the chest leads normally take place during the upstroke. The downstroke of the R merely represents the time it takes for the taut galvanometer wire to return to the midline with no electric current flowing. In heart strain, delay in depolarization results in voltage changes even during the downstroke, so that from the peak of the R down to the base line, a longer than normal time elapses. This downward stroke, as indicated above, is termed the intrinsicoid deflection, and ordinarily its measurement is not performed. When the intrinsicoid deflection is slurred in the chest leads, however, the delay characteristic of hypertrophy is obvious without measurement.

The ventricular activation time (VAT) is the time taken for an impulse to traverse the myocardium from endocardial to epicardial surface and is reflected in the measurement of the time interval from the beginning of Q to the peak of R and is prolonged when the onset of the intrinsicoid deflection is delayed.

(4) In addition to the QRS and T wave changes the ST segment is frequently below the isoelectric line.

With left ventricular strain, high R and negative ST and T occur in left ventricular positions, i.e. V5 and V6, and this is illustrated in Fig. 28.

RIGHT VENTRICULAR HYPERTROPHY

This is usually associated with right axis deviation and the diagnostic electrocardiographic signs are:—

(1) Increased voltage of the R wave over the right ventricular

leads and altered R/S ratios, the S waves over the left precordial leads being greater than normal.

(2) A QR pattern may be present in lead AVR. This may be due to (a) marked clockwise rotation so that the left ventricle faces lead AVR or (b) the possibility that in right ventricular hypertrophy lead AVR faces a portion of the right ventricle and consequently faces the depolarization wave more directly. The diagnosis, of

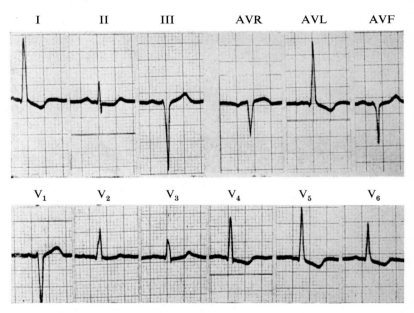

FIG. 28. Left ventricular hypertrophy ('strain pattern').

right ventricular hypertrophy, therefore, may be made when the QRS complex of AVR is more positive than negative, and about 50 per cent of all patients with an R as high as 4 mm have right ventricular strain, no matter how negative the Q or S may be. Moreover, a positive T in AVR is abnormal and may indicate right strain.

(3) Delayed onset of the intrinsicoid deflection over the right ventricular leads.

(4) Depression of the ST segment and inversion of the T wave

over the right ventricular positions, i.e. V1 and V2, but here a normal negative T wave must be differentiated.

Right ventricular hypertrophy or 'strain' is illustrated in Fig. 29 and may be seen in pulmonary embolism and overtransfusion.

BUNDLE BRANCH BLOCK

This condition, which may be permanent, intermittent or transient, is due to a block in one of the branches of the bundle of His. When the QRS complex is 0·12 second or more, complete bundle branch

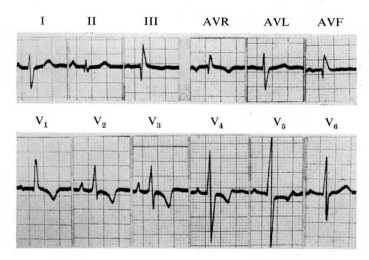

FIG. 29. Right ventricular hypertrophy ('strain pattern') P. pulmonale in leads V2 and 3.

block is present. If between 0·10 and 0·12 second, incomplete bundle branch block may be said to exist. Bundle branch block is primarily an electrocardiographic diagnosis and may occur in clinically normal hearts.

Bundle branch block is divided into right and left block. In typical block, the T wave is opposite to the main part of the QRS complex, but in atypical block the converse holds. Bundle branch block will be further discussed under disorders of cardiac rhythm.

4

ALTERATIONS MAINLY AFFECTING THE
ST SEGMENT AND T WAVE

MYOCARDIAL INFARCTION

This probably results in three physiologically abnormal zones. The centre is the zone of necrosis (electrically inert), the surrounding area is the zone of injury (electro-negative), wherein either healing or necrosis will result, and around this is the zone of ischaemia. Healthy tissue is electro-positive. The necrotic centre affects the tracing in two major ways: (a) the R will be small or absent when the electrode subtends necrotic tissue, because depolarization is minimal or absent and (b) there will be a prominent, often wide, Q wave, because the dead tissue presents an open window to the electrode which is now electrically directly on the septum, or into the cavity of the heart.

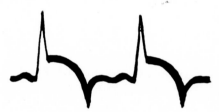

FIG. 30. The Pardee curve.

The second, or zone of injury, causes the ST interval to be elevated if the electrode is directly over the area, or depressed if more remote resulting in a depressed or elevated base line respectively (Schamroth 1961).

The classical 'Current of Injury' (the Pardee curve) is illustrated in Fig. 30 and it is on these raised ST segments that the diagnosis of infarction must be based.

The third or ischaemic zone causes inversion of the T wave.

Thus there are four changes: (1) small or absent R (2) deep Q (3) positive or negative ST and (4) inverted T.

A full thickness acute infarction of the anterior wall, presents all these changes in the precordial leads and this is shown in Fig. 31. Distinct alterations do not occur in posterior infarction because the active electrode is too remote, but depressed ST segments should make one investigate posterior infarction in the other leads, particularly leads II and III, AVF and the oesophageal lead. It should be suspected when there is a deep Q wave and an inverted T wave in leads II, III and AVF.

The right ventricle is very rarely involved.

Very low or absent R, elevated ST and depressed T over positions V5 and V6 indicate lateral wall infarction; over position V2 or V3

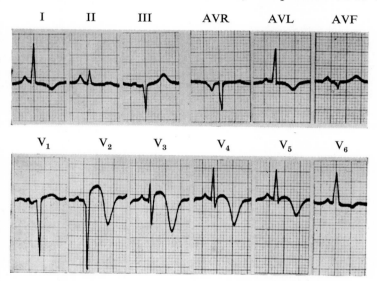

FIG. 31. Diffuse anterior myocardial infarction in a hypertensive patient.

or possibly V1 also, septal infarction and over position AVL high antero-lateral infarction.

In old infarctions, the ST usually returns to the isoelectric base in a week or two, but the other changes remain for months or years.

In the standard leads, elevations of ST occur rapidly after anterior infarction in lead I. As the infarction becomes older, the ST descends towards the base line, but it carries the negative T with it in a characteristic equilimb curve likened to a bird in flight, the final part of the QRS complex going downwards into the initial segment of the negative T with a convexity directed upward. A Q in lead I occurs in anterior infarction, but the R is not too much affected. Thus a Q and a negative T in lead I, with an isoelectric ST indicates an older infarction. This is abbreviated as Q_1T_1.

Where Q_3T_3 occurs, posterior infarction is a possibility, but in lead III it may be a normal finding. If the ST segment is elevated more than 1 mm, a diagnosis of posterior infarction can be made, and if Q is wider than 0·04 second (1 mm), an old lesion exists in the presence of an isoelectric ST.

Usually old posterior infarction cannot be diagnosed positively from lead III or from the precordial leads, if Q is 0·03 second or less, as is most often the case. It is here that the unipolar augmented limb leads assist, because AVF in part faces the posterior heart. When AVF reveals an abnormal Q, there is strong presumptive evidence of posterior wall infarction whatever the standard leads show. Perhaps of most significance here is a Q longer than 0·04 second in AVF, whether or not it is deep.

If an infarct involves only the outer third of the myocardium, no ECG changes occur, for this zone is electrically silent.

In the interpretation of ST elevations or depressions, the ST segment is compared with the T–P interval following rather than with the PR portion of the base line preceding it. That part of the tracing between the end of the T wave and the beginning of the next P wave is considered the isoelectric level and forms the base line for determining displacement of the ST segment.

PERICARDITIS

The ECG pattern of pericarditis which causes injury to the subepicardial surface of the heart is best observed in the precordial leads and is characterized by widespread elevation of the ST segments, which maintain their normal upward concavity, and the absence of abnormal Q waves. These do not appear since the injury to the heart muscle is superficial. Inverted symmetrical T waves develop after the ST segment returns to the base line. Low voltage of the QRS complexes in all leads may also be observed and is due to the fact that the electrical currents in the heart are short-circuited through the pericardial fluid and thickened pericardium.

Fig. 32 illustrates the characteristic precordial lead pattern in acute diffuse pericarditis.

MYOCARDIAL ISCHAEMIA

This causes injury to the subendocardial surface of the heart.

The classical ECG signs are ST depression and T wave flattening or inversion in leads facing the surface of the heart but leads facing the cavities (usually AVR) will show the current of injury with raised ST segments.

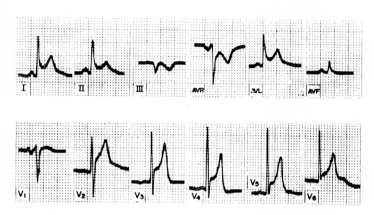

FIG. 32. Acute pericarditis pattern.

Myocardial ischaemia may be seen in the following conditions:

(1) arteriosclerosis of the coronary arteries, e.g. secondary to diabetes mellitis and myxoedema

(2) left ventricular hypertrophy

(3) aortic stenosis

(4) syphilitic aortitis

(5) pulmonary hypertension secondary to mitral stenosis or chronic diffuse pulmonary disease

(6) polycythaemia

(7) collagen diseases involving the coronary arteries, e.g. Buerger's disease

(8) anoxaemia, e.g. carbon monoxide poisoning

(9) hyperthyroidism
(10) rapid paroxysmal arrhythmias
(11) hypotension associated with severe haemorrhage
(12) hypotensive anaesthesia.
Myocardial ischaemia is illustrated in Fig. 33 and Fig. 80.

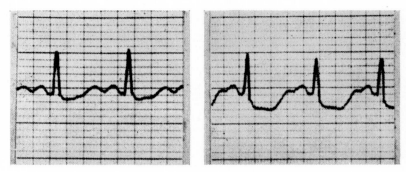

FIG. 33. Tracing on the left illustrates moderate and tracing on the right gross myocardial ischaemia.

ALTERATIONS IN THE U WAVE

While the U wave appears to have no special significance abnormal large U waves may be seen in hypokalaemia, during digitalis and quinidine therapy and in left ventricular hypertrophy, and inversion of the U wave may occur during myocardial infarction and/or ischaemia and in hyperkalaemia. Prominent U waves may also be associated with hyperventilation (Rollason & Parkes 1957).

DISORDERS OF RHYTHM

The ECG is most helpful and precise in detecting disorders of cardiac rhythm.

SINUS ARRHYTHMIA

This is a physiological arrhythmia where the record reveals a periodic acceleration of the heart. It is usually associated with the two phases of respiration; during inspiration there is lessened vagal activity with quickening of impulse formation in the SA node while during expiration there is increased vagal activity with slowing of the impulse formation.

Sinus arrhythmia is normal in children and young adults and is usually abolished by atropine and by general anaesthesia, but it may reappear during controlled respiration.

Sinus arrhythmia is illustrated in Fig. 34.

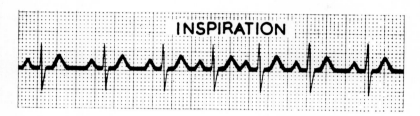

FIG. 34. Sinus arrythmia.

PATHOLOGICAL ARRHYTHMIAS

These may be classified as follows:

HEART BLOCK

    (1) Sino-atrial.
    (2) Atrio-ventricular.
        (a) 1st degree.
        (b) 2nd ,,
        (c) 3rd ,,
    (3) Bundle branch block.

ECTOPIC RHYTHM

    (1) Extrasystoles.
        (a) Atrial.
        (b) Nodal.
        (c) Ventricular.
    (2) Paroxysmal tachycardia.
        (a) Atrial.
            (i) tachycardia
            (ii) flutter
            (iii) fibrillation.

(b) Nodal (unimportant).
(c) Ventricular.
   (i) tachycardia
   (ii) fibrillation.

As far as the atrial arrhythmias are concerned Prinzmetal (1950) has shown that they depend upon the presence and behaviour of an irritable focus in atrial muscle. The type of arrhythmia produced depends on the rate of discharge of impulses from the ectopic focus. If the rate is slow, atrial extrasystoles result, but rates of 110 to 250 produce atrial tachycardia, rates of 260 to 340 atrial flutter, and rates of 400 to 600 atrial fibrillation. As the AV node can rarely transmit impulses faster than 210–20 per minute, physiological heart block results.

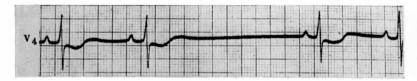

Fig. 35. Sino-atrial block. The PP interval that contains the pause is double the PP interval of the beats displaying normal sinus rhythm. A longer pause would indicate sinus arrest.

HEART BLOCK

This is a condition in which there is defective conduction in some part of the heart.

1. *Sino-atrial block*

Here the block is produced within the substance of the SA node, and the impulse has difficulty in getting out to activate the rest of the heart. It commonly results in the dropping of an entire PQRST complex. If alternate beats are dropped the heart rate is exactly half the normal. The condition is usually due to increased vagal tone acting on a susceptible SA node and can be abolished by intravenous atropine. Sino-atrial block is illustrated in Fig. 35.

2. Atrio-ventricular block

Here the whole bundle of His is damaged and changes occur in the following order:

(a) Delayed AV conduction. This is reflected in a prolongation of the PR interval which exceeds 0·2 second. This is referred to as first degree heart block and is illustrated in Fig. 36.

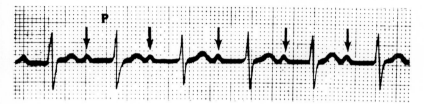

FIG. 36. First degree heart block.

(b) Failure of occasional and then of a larger proportion of the atrial impulses to reach the ventricles. The ventricles then respond to every second, third or fourth impulse from the SA node. This is referred to as second degree heart block.

A 2:1 heart block is illustrated in Fig. 37. Here the P waves are regularly spaced, but are twice as numerous as the ventricular impulses.

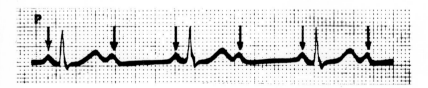

FIG. 37. Second degree (2 : 1) heart block.

Another form of second degree heart block is referred to as Wenckebach's phenomenon. The PR interval is usually normal at the onset of a cycle and gradually increases at each successive beat until the P wave is not conducted. This is illustrated in Fig. 38.

First and second degree heart block is referred to as partial heart block.

(c) Complete or third degree heart block. Here none of the atrial impulses reach the ventricles and so the beats of atria and ventricles are completely dissociated, bearing no relationship whatever to one another. The ventricles beat with an independent rhythm, and at a slower rate—usually less than 40 per minute. The independent ventricular beats arise from the most rhythmic part of the ventricle,

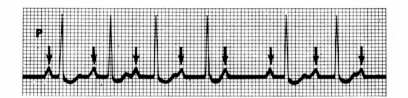

FIG. 38. Second degree heart block (Wenckebach's phenomenon).

usually the region of the bundle below the site of the block. The excitation process, therefore, reaches the two ventricles along the normal channel of the two branches of the bundle. The ventricular complex is quite normal in character. This is illustrated in Fig. 39.

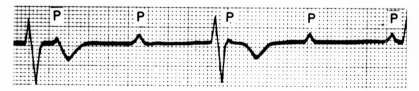

FIG. 39. Third degree (complete) heart block.

If the ventricular pacemaker is located in the bundle branches or in the ventricular muscle (idioventricular rhythm), the QRS complexes are wide, slurred and notched, and have the characteristics of ventricular premature beats.

Widened and slurred QRS complexes may also, together with absent P waves, constitute the tracing of the 'dying heart' which frequently precedes asystole or ventricular fibrillation.

3. *Bundle branch block*
This was referred to on page 29.

Right bundle branch block. When the right bundle is blocked, the sequence of depolarization is:—

(1) Depolarization of the septum from left to right (the right side is activated below the point of block by the stimulus from the left), resulting in a R wave.

(2) Depolarization of the free wall of the left ventricle results in a S wave.

(3) Depolarization of the free wall of the right ventricle resulting in a R^1 wave. The electrical events on the left side of the heart are normal.

The diagnostic electrocardiographic signs are:—

(1) QRS widened to 0·12 second or more

(2) Late onset of the intrinsicoid deflection over the right ventricular leads (V1 and V2)

(3) Increased amplitude of the R^1 wave in the right precordial leads

(4) Depression of the ST segment and inversion of the T wave (typical block) over the right precordial leads. If the T wave is upright, it is referred to as atypical bundle branch block

(5) Left ventricular precordial leads show a slurred broad S wave due to the late right ventricular depolarization

(6) A QR pattern in lead AVR

(7) Frequently a broad S wave in lead I

Right bundle branch block is illustrated in Fig. 40.

It is sometimes found in a heart which is otherwise normal. It then may have no serious significance.

In disease, right bundle branch block is associated with conditions producing great dilatation of the right ventricle, such as atrial septal defect where it occurs in partial or complete form in 95 per cent of cases.

It may also be associated with pulmonary embolism, coronary artery, hypertensive and valvular heart disease.

Left bundle branch block. When the left bundle is blocked the sequence of depolarization is:—

(1) Depolarization of the septum is from right to left so that the

left side of the septum below the point of the block is activated by the stimulus from the right

(2) Depolarization of the free wall of the right ventricle

(3) Depolarization of the free wall of the left ventricle. The electrical events in the right side of the heart are normal.

The diagnostic electrocardiographic signs are:—

(1) QRS widened to 0·12 second or more

(2) Late onset of the intrinsicoid deflection in leads over the left ventricle (V4–V6)

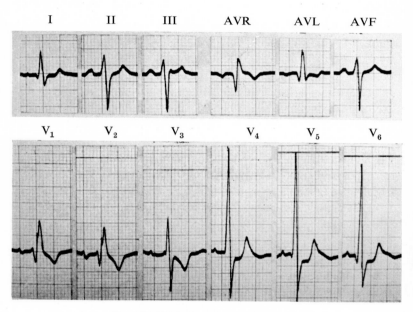

FIG. 40. Right bundle branch block.

(3) Depressed ST segments and inverted T waves over the left chest leads

(4) Right ventricular precordial leads show a slurred broad S wave due to the late left ventricular depolarization and the ST segments may be slightly elevated.

Left bundle branch block is illustrated in Fig. 41.

Very rarely left bundle branch block may be present in a clinically normal heart. It is seen most commonly in coronary artery disease, hypertensive heart disease and aortic stenosis.

Wolff-Parkinson-White syndrome. This is characterized by a wide

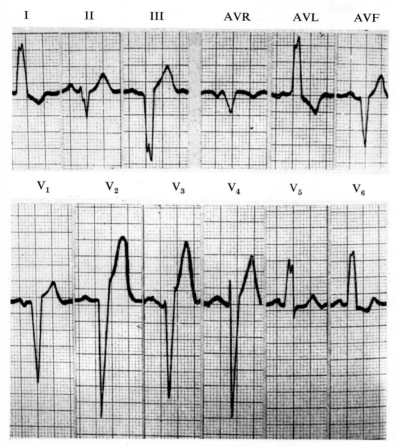

FIG. 41. Left bundle branch block.

QRS complex (0·11–0·14 second) and a short PR interval (0·10 second or less). This is illustrated in Fig. 42.

The syndrome usually occurs in healthy young persons who have a tendency to recurrent attacks of cardiac arrhythmia and in itself is not indicative of organic heart disease. It must be distinguished

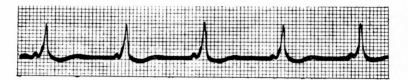

FIG. 42. Wolff-Parkinson-White Syndrome.

from bundle branch block. Although the PR interval is short the PS interval is normal.

ECTOPIC RHYTHM

1. *Extrasystoles*

(a) *Atrial.* If the atrium is stimulated during diastole after its refractory period has passed, it responds with a premature contraction. An impulse is transmitted to the ventricles which contract too. The P wave is usually abnormal in configuration, (e.g. inverted or isoelectric) and the PR interval shortens, but the succeeding ventricular complex is usually normal. The next atrial impulse arising in the SA node appears after a pause equal to the normal diastolic period or a little in excess of it. An atrial extrasystole is illustrated in Fig. 43. When the atrial beat is so premature that the

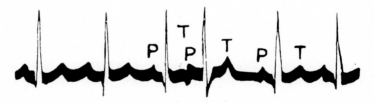

FIG. 43. Atrial extrasystole.

ventricles are in refractory state they fail to respond. Atrial extrasystoles are common during cardiac surgery and appear to have no special significance.

The phenomenon of wandering pacemaker refers to a shift in origin of the stimulus between the SA and AV nodes and is characterized by changes in the form of the P waves and by changing PR intervals from beat to beat in the same lead. It is sometimes referred to as a shifting or sliding nodal rhythm. Fig. 44 illustrates a wandering pacemaker with excursions limited between the SA and upper AV node and a wandering pacemaker in the AV node.

(b) *Nodal.* Here the P wave, which is usually deformed, is placed shortly before or after, or may coincide with a ventricular complex. The beat occurs prematurely and is followed by a compensatory pause. It can be precipitated by increased vagal activity.

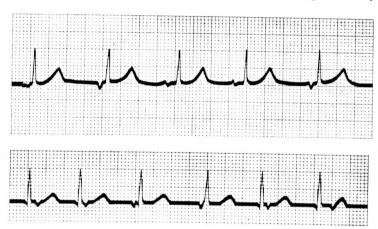

FIG. 44. *Upper tracing:* Wandering pacemaker with excursions limited between the SA and upper AV node.
   Lower tracing: Wandering pacemaker in the AV node.

When the ectopic focus remains in the AV node, nodal rhythm is produced. There are three types of nodal rhythm depending on whether the impulse arises in the upper, mid or lower portion of the AV node. When the impulse arises in the upper portion of the node, the P wave falls just before the QRS complex and is referred to as superior nodal or coronary sinus rhythm. When the impulse arises in the mid portion of the node, the P wave is buried in the QRS complex and as a consequence is not visible. This is referred to as mid nodal or just nodal rhythm. When the impulse arises in the lower portion of the node, the P wave follows the QRS complex and is referred to as inferior nodal rhythm.

Nodal rhythm is frequently seen during anaesthesia and appears to have no special significance. It is usually associated with increased vagal tone. It may also occur during stimulation of the atrial musculature during surgery and during cardiac catheterization. Nodal rhythm is illustrated in Fig. 45.

(c) *Ventricular.* If the ventricle is stimulated during diastole after its refractory period has passed, it also responds with a premature contraction. The ventricular complex is abnormal and is not preceded by a P wave. The next P wave is usually 'buried' within this ventricular complex. The excitation process which arises in the new focus spreads radially over the surface of the ventricular

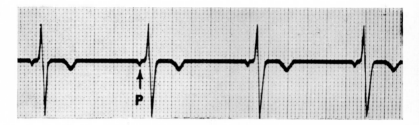

FIG. 45. Nodal rhythm.

muscle in all directions: it also penetrates the ventricular wall to reach the endocardium and so invades the Punkinje tissue which transmits the excitation process rapidly over its own side of the heart. The same change occurs later in the contralateral ventricle. As the time taken for the excitation process to affect the whole of both ventricles is prolonged, the QRS will exceed 0·12 second in duration; as the pattern of invasion is abnormal, the deflections of the QRS will be abnormal in appearance. The pattern of repolarization is also altered with consequent changes in the ST segment and the T wave. There is no isoelectric portion of the ST segment and the T wave takes off from a level above or below the isoelectric line and usually has a direction opposite to that of the main deflection of the QRS complex. A ventricular extrasystole is illustrated in Fig. 46. When the ectopic focus originates in the right ventricle, the QRS deflection resembles a left bundle branch block pattern

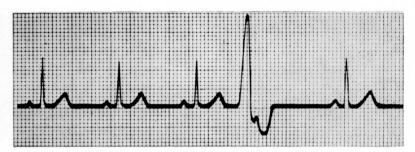

FIG. 46. Ventricular extrasystole.

as seen in the right precordial leads and when it originates in the left ventricle the QRS resembles right bundle branch block pattern as seen in the right precordial leads. If ventricular extrasystoles become frequent, they interfere with the efficiency of the circulation as the output produced by a premature beat is less than normal because the ventricle has not had time to fill. Multifocal ventricular

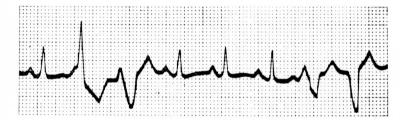

FIG. 47. Multifocal ventricular extrasystoles.

extrasystoles (Fig. 47) are usually ominous and may be followed by ventricular fibrillation (Fig. 48).

2. *Paroxysmal tachycardia.* This term is applied to attacks of rapid heart action where ventricular contraction responds to regular impulses arising in a focus removed from the SA node, the rate may be as slow as 100 per minute or as rapid as 210 or even faster in infants. Three forms of paroxysmal tachycardia are recognized according to whether the ectopic focus of stimulus formation is situated in the atrium, AV node or ventricle. The essential characteristics of all types of tachycardia are:

5

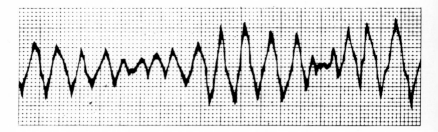

FIG. 48. Ventricular fibrillation.

1. They begin suddenly
2. The first beat is a premature one
3. The beats are absolutely regular
4. They terminate suddenly
5. Carotid sinus pressure or pressure on the eyeball may change the rate or stop the paroxysm completely.

(a) *Atrial.* (i) Atrial tachycardia. Here there is a rapid succession of abnormal P waves. The fact that the impulse initiating atrial contraction commences in a focus removed from the SA node explains the inversion or other deformity of the P wave. Often the P waves appear to be unaltered but when they are compared with those in a tracing obtained before or after the paroxysm, it will be seen that during the attack they differed from the normal for that individual. The ventricular complexes following the P wave are usually normal. Paroxysmal atrial tachycardia is illustrated in Fig. 49.

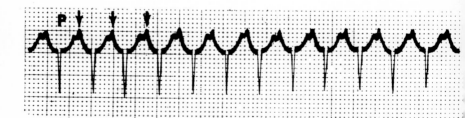

FIG. 49. Paroxysmal atrial tachycardia.

(ii) Atrial flutter. Here the P waves are absolutely regular in rhythm. They are characterized by a rapid upstroke and a more gradual downstroke and by the absence of any isoelectric interval between the waves. The waves occur in rapid succession, usually 260–340 per minute, but occasionally as much as 400 per minute. The ratio between atrial and ventricular complexes is commonly 2:1 as a physiological heart block occurs but the ventricle may respond less frequently so that a 4:1 response is not unusual. When the ratio is 1:1 the tracing is difficult to distinguish from one of paroxysmal atrial tachycardia, but in the latter condition the rate is usually less than 210. Fig. 50 illustrates a case of atrial flutter.

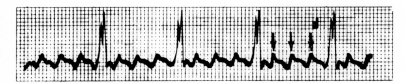

FIG. 50. Atrial flutter.

Digitalis often converts flutter to fibrillation and with the cessation of its administration a normal rhythm may result.

Atrial flutter may be precipitated by cardiac catheterization and other cardiac manoeuvres.

(iii) Atrial fibrillation. Here the tracing shows no true P waves which are replaced by oscillations called 'f' waves, which are irregular in shape, at a rate of 400–600 per minute. The ventricular complexes are usually normal but they occur at irregular intervals which is a characteristic feature giving rise to the typical irregular irregularity of the pulse. Exceptionally, the pulse may be slow and completely regular when complete heart block is associated with atrial fibrillation.

Atrial fibrillation is illustrated in Fig. 51.

This arrhythmia occurs most commonly in rheumatic mitral valvular disease, coronary artery disease and hyperthyroidism. It may also occur in clinically normal hearts and in association with cardiotomy and hypothermia.

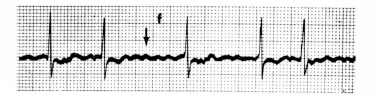

FIG. 51. Atrial fibrillation.

(b) *Nodal.* Here the P wave is usually inverted and the PR interval shortened. The P wave precedes or follows or, occasionally, coincides with the ventricular complex which is usually normal in configuration. Nodal tachycardia is illustrated in Fig. 52.

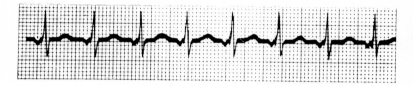

FIG. 52. Nodal tachycardia.

When the rate is rapid it is impossible to differentiate nodal from atrial tachycardia and in such instances the term supraventricular tachycardia is applied.

(c) *Ventricular.* (i) Ventricular tachycardia. Here the P waves are lost in the large excursions of the ventricular complexes which have a wide and notched appearance. They are regular in rhythm and are followed by large secondary T waves which are directed opposite to the main deflection of the QRS complex. Paroxysmal ventricular tachycardia is illustrated in Fig. 53.

This arrhythmia may precede ventricular fibrillation and it may occur after coronary occlusion.

(ii) Ventricular fibrillation. Ventricular fibrillation (Fig. 48) occurs when individual myocardial fibres are out of phase. Excitation then spreads from one fibre which contracts to another which is resting. This excitation is effective only when the refractory period is abnormally short.

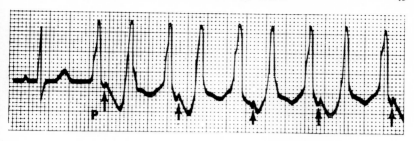

FIG. 53. Paroxysmal ventricular tachycardia.

Under normal conditions the long refractory period of cardiac muscle as compared with that of skeletal muscle protects it from fibrillation.

COMBINED MECHANISM

It should be realized that more than one arrhythmia may occur simultaneously as in the case instanced above, where atrial fibrillation occurs in the presence of complete AV block.

ARTEFACTS

These may be grouped into (a) those common to electrocardiography wherever it is performed and (b) those peculiar to electrocardiography in the operating theatre.

(a) COMMON ARTEFACTS

(i) *Muscle tremor.* It is important for the conscious patient to be warm and relaxed when the record is taken as any muscle tremor such as that produced by shivering can alter the tracing. This type of interference is illustrated in Fig. 54. Electrodes strapped on too tightly may also produce muscle tremor. They should be held just tightly enough so that the electrode does not slide over the skin when moved gently by hand.

(ii) *Movement of the patient.* Movement on the part of the patient with the associated contraction of skeletal muscle causes sudden changes in the current conducted through the galvanometer resulting in sudden deflections. In addition, movement of the subject disturbs the contacts of the electrodes on the body which, in turn,

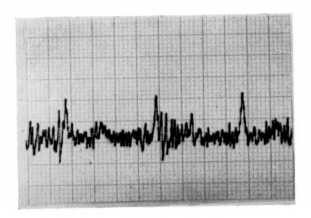

FIG. 54. Muscle tremor.

causes changes in the resistance between the skin and the electrodes resulting in movements of the galvanometer string. These effects are illustrated in Fig. 55.

(iii) *Overshooting*. This occurs when the galvanometer string is loose and results in an abnormally high amplitude of the deflections with slurring and widening of the complexes as seen in Fig. 56.

(iv) *Shifting of the base (isoelectric) line*. This is often due to cutaneous currents, polarization of the electrodes, variations in

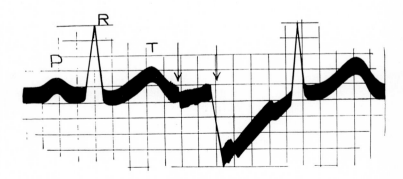

FIG. 55. Shifting of the galvanometer string.

cutaneous resistance or wires conducting electricity in the vicinity of the recording leads and is illustrated in Fig. 57.

(v) *Loose contacts.* These may occur in any part of the circuit and produce sudden shifting of the base line as shown in Fig. 58.

(vi) *Inadequate earthing.* When the patient or the machine is not properly earthed alternating current may produce gross interfer-

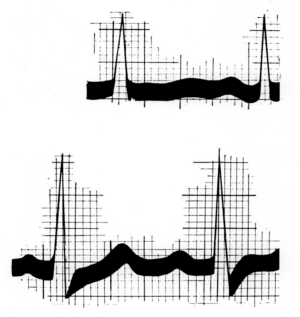

FIG. 56. Overshooting produced by a loose galvanometer string is seen in the lower tracing.

ence at the rate of 50 times a second in 50 cycle alternating current as shown in Fig. 59.

(vii) *Incorrectly connected leads.* When abnormal wave forms for a particular lead present incorrect placement of the leads should be suspected. For example, if the right and left arm leads are reversed, simulating dextrocardia, lead I becomes the mirror image of itself, and leads II and III become reversed as do also leads AVR and AVL. This is illustrated in Fig. 60.

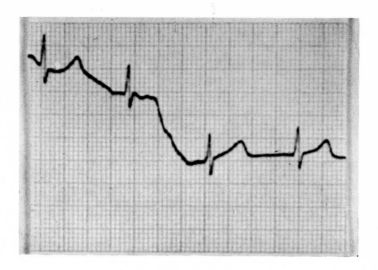

FIG. 57. Shifting of the base line.

(viii) *Inaccurate standardization and damping effects*. Over or under standardisation will result in an abnormal increase or decrease in the voltage of the complexes respectively. Proper standardisation exists when 1 mV produces a deflection of 1 cm (Fig. 61A). If the machine is overdamped the mV deflection will be distorted by under shooting (Fig. 61B). This may result in

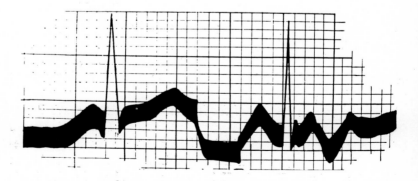

FIG. 58. Sudden shifting of the base line.

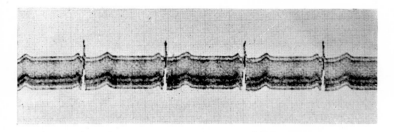

FIG. 59. 50 cycle interference ('hum').

artificially depressed or elevated ST segments as well as other distortions. If the machine is underdamped the standardizing deflection will be distorted by overshooting (Fig. 61c). This may cause excessive amplitude of the R waves and other distortions.

(b) ARTEFACTS PECULIAR TO THE OPERATING THEATRE
These will be discussed in Chapter V.

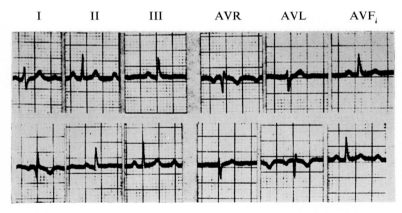

FIG. 60. *Upper tracing:* normal ECG picture.
    Lower tracing: Leads incorrectly connected. Right and left arm leads reversed. Lead I is mirror image of itself, leads II and III are reversed, as are also leads AVR and AVL. (Compare with Fig. 21 which illustrates the ECG in dextrocardia.)

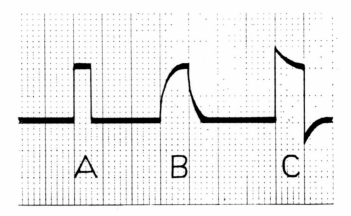

FIG. 61. (A) Correct standardization (B) overdamping (C) under-damping.

CHAPTER IV

THE EFFECT OF ANAESTHETIC AGENTS, ELECTROLYTE IMBALANCE AND CARDIAC DRUGS ON THE ECG

PREMEDICATION

MORPHIA AND SCOPOLAMINE

Kurtz et al (1936) studied premedication with morphia and scopolamine and found a tendency to produce small changes in the QRS complex and T wave together with slight ST segment depression and an increase in pulse rate.

Apart, however, from the sinus tachycardia usually produced by such drugs as atropine and chlorpromazine, routine premedication appears to have no significant effect on the ECG. As the main coronary inflow occurs in diastole, drugs which increase the heart rate shorten diastole and should be avoided in patients with hyperthyroidism and cardiac disease except those with heart block.

Apprehension and anxiety are common causes of tachycardia and should be dealt with by appropriate reassurance and sedation.

ATROPINE

In the conscious and fit subject atropine may produce a tachycardia or a bradycardia (Rollason 1957; Morton & Thomas 1958). It may also produce a supra-ventricular arrhythmia, such as nodal rhythm and nodal extrasystoles (Averill & Lamb 1959; Jones et al 1961), but in the presence of adrenaline, CO_2 retention and potassium imbalance it may precipitate ventricular fibrillation. Atropine is thus a drug the anaesthetist should treat with respect, particularly when administered intravenously. There is evidence in the dog that it increases the oxygen consumption of the myocardium more than the coronary flow (Scott et al 1959). It is important to administer atropine prior to ECT as otherwise cardiac asystole may occur during the clonic phase of the convulsion (Dobkin 1959), and Clement (1962) recommends that the atropine be given intravenously 75 seconds prior to the shock but ECG changes have been noted following the too rapid injection of this drug (Gottlieb & Sweet 1963).

CHLORPROMAZINE

This also produces a tachycardia in some patients but it appears to increase the coronary flow and sinus rhythm is usual. There may be a slight depression up to 1 mm of the ST segment but this can be produced by tachycardia alone. Injected intravenously into normal man in a dose of 25 mg chlorpromazine has been shown to check the development of the ECG signs of hypoxia produced by the inhalation of an atmosphere containing only 6 per cent oxygen (Szabo *et al* 1957).

BARBITURATES

Provided respiratory depression and CO_2 retention are avoided, these appear to have no significant effects on the ECG of normal man.

Thiopentone may cause an increase in the height of the P wave but this is probably related to an increase in the pulse rate and a fall in BP rather than to the drug per se (Rollason & Hough 1958).

Henderson *et al* (1958) found that buthalitone produced a greater prolongation of the QTc interval than thiopentone and suggested the QTc interval may be an index of the cardiotoxicity of a drug.

RELAXANTS

Apart from the tachycardia produced by gallamine triethiodide suxamethonium appears to be the only relaxant which produces significant changes in the ECG pattern provided anoxia and CO_2 retention are avoided. This relaxant drug, when given intravenously, can not only produce a sinus bradycardia but also a disturbance of rhythm in both children and adults. These effects have been recorded by a number of investigators (Philips 1954; Johnstone 1955; Leigh *et al* 1957; Martin 1958; Barreto 1960; Craythorne *et al* 1960; Bickman & Halldin 1960; Lupprian & Churchill-Davidson 1960; Foster 1961; Sagarminaga & Wynands 1963). The nature of the arrhythmia is a depression of excitation and conduction of the cardiac impulse producing changes in the P wave, PR interval, QRS complex and ventricular standstill up to 16 seconds. These changes are illustrated in Fig. 62. A case of prolonged cardiac arrest following an injection of suxamethonium in a severely burned patient has been reported by Allen *et al* (1961) and by Bush *et al* (1962). Both the bradycardia and arrhythmia associated with suxamethonium can be antagonized by the intravenous injection of atropine, and it is the author's practice to give this drug after an injection of suxamethonium if the heart rate falls to 40 per minute or below, and/or if the rhythm becomes irregular. Atropine gr.1/100 diluted to 4 cc with normal saline should be immediately available for use prior to the induction of anaesthesia.

INHALATIONAL AGENTS

The effect of these agents on the ECG varies.

Some, like nitrous oxide, in the presence of adequate oxygenation have no effect whereas others, like chloroform, can produce profound disturbances.

The changes are usually due to either vagal stimulation or sympathetic overactivity. Vagal stimulation produces a bradycardia with reduction in the height of the P wave. If the stimulus is marked partial or complete heart block or even asystole may occur. Sympathetic overactivity, on the other hand, produces a tachycardia, with an increase in the height of the P wave, and occasional ventricular extrasystoles. If the stimulus is marked the ventricular extrasystoles become more frequent and may develop into multifocal ventricular extrasystoles, which may be the precursor of ventricular fibrillation.

1. CHLOROFORM

Levy (1913, 1914) postulated ventricular fibrillation as the cause of sudden death during induction with chloroform in the cat, and the classical work of Hill (1932a, b) in man, demonstrated multifocal ventricular tachycardia in about 50 per cent of cases during induction and that the arrhythmia disappeared as anaesthesia was deepened. Goodman & Gilman (1955) suggest that the irritant effect of the vapour on the respiratory passages stimulates cardiac reflexes initiated from the brain stem through the spinal cord and stellate ganglion to the heart by way of the cardiac sympathetic nerves to cause tachycardia and ventricular extrasystoles. The liberation of endogenous adrenaline from the suprarenal by fear, pain, hypoxia or CO_2 retention, or the injection of adrenaline by the surgeon may act on a chloroform sensitized myocardium to precipitate a dangerous or even fatal ventricular arrhythmia. The onset of multifocal ventricular extrasystoles should constitute a warning to the anaesthetist to stop the administration of chloroform and ventilate his patient with pure oxygen. Vagal inhibition may also be a cause of death during induction with chloroform. A period of breath holding when using the open drop method of administration could result in the build up of an irritant concentration of the vapour resulting in reflex asystole when the patient decides to start breathing again (pulmocardiac reflex). To avoid these hazards, chloroform should be administered through an accurately calibrated vaporizer, such as a Chlorotec, and the patient should be adequately premedicated and induced with an intravenous barbiturate.

2. DI-ETHYL-ETHER

From a practical point of view, ether is probably still the safest of the inhalational agents, although the deliberate forced inflation of a high concentration of vapour has resulted in cardiac standstill This is more likely to occur when the larynx has been paralysed by a relaxant.

Ether may cause alteration in the height of the P wave and a wandering pacemaker, but these are of no particular significance and may occur under any type of anaesthesia. Vinyl-ether and methyl-N-propyl ether behave in a similar way and do not sensitize the myocardium to the effects of adrenaline.

3. ETHYL CHLORIDE

This agent should be treated with the same respect as chloroform for its administration carries similar risks. Fortunately, it is used simply for induction, so that if this can be achieved without vagal inhibition, the ventricular extrasystoles associated with deep ethyl chloride anaesthesia are not seen. Because of its greater safety factor vinyl ether has replaced ethyl chloride in the North American continent.

4. TRICHLORETHYLENE

Almost every known form of cardiac arrhythmia has been reported during anaesthesia with this agent, but as it is now generally used only as an analgesic supplement, cardiac arrhythmias in these light levels are not so frequently observed. Orth (1958), however, found ECG evidence of irregularities in about two-thirds of patients.

In higher concentrations, trichlorethylene produces tachypnoea which results in CO_2 retention, but this and the associated ventricular arrhythmias can be abolished by the intravenous injection of pethidine (Johnstone 1951).

Being a halogen-containing compound, it sensitizes the heart to adrenaline.

5. HALOTHANE

The vagal effects of this drug on the heart are common and if the pulse rate falls below 40 per minute in the presence of adequate oxygenation and CO_2 elimination, it can be corrected by injecting 0·15 mg (1/400 gr) of atropine intravenously. Occasionally ventricular extrasystoles follow the injection of this drug.

Ventricular extrasystoles may also occur in association with hypoventilation and CO_2 retention (Millar et al 1958; Black et al 1959), but these can be prevented by hyperventilation and CO_2 absorption. Only rarely have extrasystoles of the multifocal variety been seen (Payne & Plantevin 1962).

Endotracheal intubation under halothane has been shown to produce ventricular arrhythmia (Burnap et al 1958; Delaney 1958), Gauthier et al (1962) and Robson & Sheridan (1957) showed that stretching the anal sphincter could produce a similar effect.

Brindle et al (1957) and Millar et al (1958) demonstrated that the use of adrenaline could induce ventricular extrasystoles and ventricular tachycardia during halothane anaesthesia but the author has not seen them in the presence of small amounts (0·15–0·35 mg) of subcutaneously injected adrenaline when the patient has been well oxygenated, hyperventilated to eliminate CO_2 retention, and premedicated with perphenazine. The intravenous injection of adrenaline, however, particularly in the presence of hypoxia and CO_2 retention, may well precipitate ventricular fibrillation. In this connection it is of interest to note that halothane anaesthesia has been used successfully for the surgical removal of a phaeochromo-cytoma (Rollason 1963) and for open cardiac surgery during which intracardiac adrenaline was used, but no ventricular tachycardia or fibrillation ensued (Orton & Morris 1959; Dawson et al 1960). Nevertheless, the intrusion of frequent ventricular extrasystoles into the ECG pattern should be regarded by the anaesthetist as a warning signal not to be ignored and it should be noted that two cases of cardiac arrest have occurred following the combination of adrenaline infiltration and halothane anaesthesia, both during reconstructive operations on the vagina (Rosen & Roe 1963).

Halothane in high concentration and in association with con-trolled respiration can produce profound hypotension resulting in either asystole or ventricular fibrillation, but the use of accurately calibrated vaporizers outside the circuit, together with the con-tinuous monitoring of BP, PR and ECG should prevent this occurring.

This agent facilitates the induction of surface hypothermia and does not appear to increase the incidence of ventricular arrhyth-mias provided the temperature does not fall below 28° C. (82·4° F.) and hyperventilation is ensured. (Rollason & Latham, 1963).

6. CYCLOPROPANE

This is the only gaseous agent which can produce serious cardiac arrhythmias.

Johnstone (1950) pointed out that ventricular arrhythmias are frequent during deep cyclopropane anaesthesia, but they can usually be prevented by adequate oxygenation. He also showed (Johnstone 1953) that these arrhythmias were frequent in the pre-sence of intramuscular adrenaline and noradrenaline, but that they could be inhibited by stimulating the pulmo-cardiac reflex with ether. Lurie et al (1958) have, however, shown that cyclopropane itself can produce ventricular arrhythmias in normal man not subjected to operation and in the presence of adequate oxygenation and CO_2 elimination. The presence of arrhythmia in these circumstances suggests a high cyclopropane concentration. Ventricular arrhythmias are common in the lighter levels of cyclopropane anaesthesia in the presence of CO_2 retention, and are further accentuated when an elevated pCO_2 is suddenly reduced and this is particularly so in the presence of the higher blood concentrations of cyclopropane. Price *et al* (1958), however, have found that bilateral stellate ganglion blockade with a local anaesthetic can render CO_2 retention relatively ineffective in producing these ventricular arrhythmias. In the patient under cyclopropane anaesthesia an injection of gallamine may precipitate a ventricular tachycardia and this relaxant should be avoided.

ADRENALINE AND NORADRENALINE

The use of adrenaline and noradrenaline can induce ventricular arrhythmias which may terminate in ventricular fibrillation during anaesthesia, with chloroform, ethyl chloride, trichlorethylene, halothane and cyclopropane, particularly if CO_2 retention is also present. It is probable that all these agents interfere with the supply or availability of energy, i.e. oxygen and glucose and the refractory period of cardiac muscle is as a consequence shortened. Some adrenolytic compounds can suppress these adrenaline induced arrhythmias and of those in current use, perphenazine appears to be the most effective. Because this drug also has good antiemetic properties, it is the author's practice to use it routinely, both in premedication and in association with methadone for sedation in the early post-operative period. When a pressor agent must be administered to patients already anaesthetized with halogenated vapours or cyclopropane mephentermine and methoxamine seem to be the safest (Benazon 1962).

PITOCIN

This drug may be used in obstetrics and the anaesthetist should eschew the use of cyclopropane in its presence, as ventricular arrhythmias terminating in ventricular fibrillation may occur.

6

NEOSTIGMINE AND ATROPINE

Jacobson *et al* (1954) studying the ECG effects of the intravenous administration of neostigmine followed by atropine during cyclopropane anaesthesia, found that neostigmine in doses of 0·5–2·0 mg produced profound disruption of AV conduction, sinus depression and sinus arrest. The injection, however, of 0·8 mg atropine resulted in marked adrenergic activity with multifocal ventricular extrasystoles and paroxysmal ventricular tachycardia.

Under ordinary conditions the muscarinic action of neostigmine predominates, but in the atropinized patient the muscarinic action is blocked and the nicotinic effect predominates, so the result is as if an adrenergic drug was administered, but the dose of atropine required to achieve this may be as high as 2–3 mg. It would, however, appear that the combined effect of neostigmine and atropine may in some patients produce sufficient adrenergic stimulation to precipitate ventricular fibrillation, particularly during cyclopropane anaesthesia, in the presence of CO_2 retention, and in states of potassium imbalance.

Johnstone (1951) showed that ventricular arrhythmias can appear within 30 seconds after the intravenous injection of atropine in patients under cyclopropane-ether anaesthesia with CO_2 retention. These arrhythmias took the form of a multifocal ventricular tachycardia in ten of the fifteen cases studied, and the view expressed by Pooler (1957) that atropine in association with CO_2 retention is the cause of the sudden deaths following the simultaneous intravenous injection of neostigmine and atropine to reverse curarization is the correct one. This view is further substantiated by the fact that sudden deaths have occurred after the injection of atropine alone, before any neostigmine was administered, at the end of operative procedures in patients with CO_2 retention, tachycardia and potassium imbalance.

In a series of 37 cases, the author observed no significant ECG changes either when atropine and neostigmine were given together or when the atropine preceded the neostigmine (Rollason 1958), but these cases had received a ganglionic blocking drug and had been well oxygenated and ventilated.

In another series of 24 cases, Riding & Robinson (1961) studied the ECG effects of atropine and neostigmine and correlated these effects with changes in acid base balance. No significant ECG changes followed the injection of atropine and changes followed the injection of neostigmine, given five minutes later, only in those cases with CO_2 retention. These changes involved most components of the ECG and included extrasystoles, heart block, gross voltage reduction and transient cardiac arrest. It was concluded that in healthy patients the heart was protected from the effects of neo-stigmine by a respiratory alkalosis.

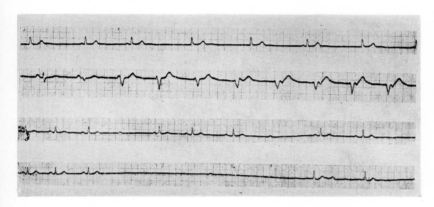

Fig. 62. *Top tracing:* Variations of the P wave.
Second tracing: Wide QRS complexes followed by inverted P waves.
Third tracing: Wenckebach's phenomenon.
Bottom tracing: Ventricular standstill.

Respiratory alkalosis, unlike respiratory acidosis, appears to produce no significant ECG changes (Rollason & Parkes 1957).

CARBON DIOXIDE

The inhalation of carbon dioxide in oxygen produces a respiratory acidosis which causes a delayed conduction within the myocardium resulting in prolongation of the PR, QRS and QT intervals (Altschule & Sulzbach 1947; McArdle 1959).

Periods of paroxysmal tachycardia and atrial extrasystoles may also be seen. It should, however, be remembered that the absence

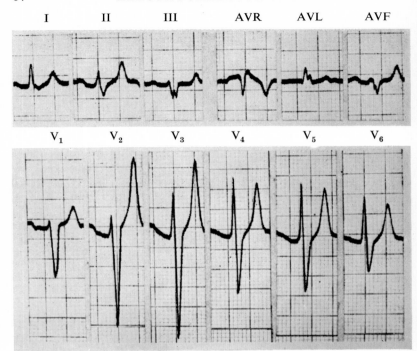

FIG. 63. Hyperkalaemia – serum K 7·6 m eq./litre – a case of uraemia.

of hypoxia and other complicating factors distinguish the dangers of inhaling carbon dioxide in oxygen from carbon dioxide accumulation occurring during anaesthesia, where in association with anoxia, electrolyte imbalance, atropine, and adrenaline, it may predispose to ventricular fibrillation.

ELECTROLYTE IMBALANCE

POTASSIUM

Hyperkalaemia. A high serum potassium may be found in patients with Addison's disease, uraemia, shock, anoxia, dehydration, severe burns, and in patients on low sodium diets. It may also be seen in those receiving massive blood transfusions and in those on a KCl drip, particularly in the presence of inadequate renal function. Hyperkalaemia is characterized initially by tall peaked T waves and these are illustrated in Fig. 63.

The sequence of ECG changes with increasing concentrations of serum potassium is illustrated diagrammatically in Fig. 64.

Hypokalaemia. A low serum potassium may be seen in patients with diabetic acidosis, primary aldosteronism, potassium losing nephritis, excessive diarrhoea, and following the excessive use of

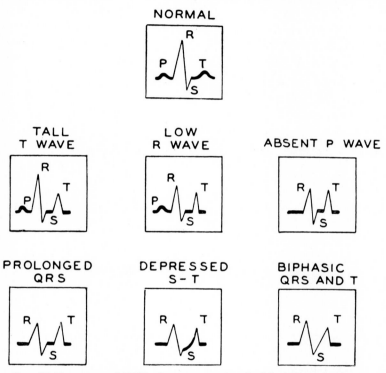

FIG. 64. Sequence of ECG changes associated with progressive hyperkalaemia. Terminal biphasic complex appears with potassium levels in the region of 10 m eq/litre.

steroids and certain diuretics. Hypokalaemia is characterized initially with prolongation of the QT interval, lowering or inversion of the T waves, and prominent U waves. These are illustrated in Fig. 65, and are best seen in leads V2 to V5.

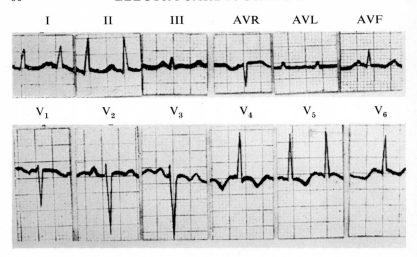

FIG. 65. Hypokalaemia – serum K 2·2 m eq/litre – a case of diabetic acidosis. Late inverted T wave and prominent U waves in almost all leads especially V2 and V5, depressed ST segments; and prolonged QT interval.

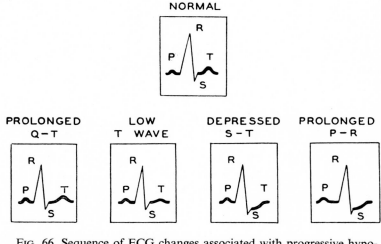

FIG. 66. Sequence of ECG changes associated with progressive hypokalaemia. Terminal prolongation of PR interval appears with potassium levels in the region of 1·5 m eq/litre.

The sequence of ECG changes with decreasing levels of serum potassium is illustrated diagrammatically in Fig. 66.

Digitalis must be used with great caution in hypokalaemic states, particularly those due to potassium depleting diuretics.

CALCIUM

Hypercalcaemia. A high serum calcium may be associated with hyperparathyroidism. The QT interval varies inversely with the calcium level of the blood and in patients with a parathyroid tumour the QT interval may be so shortened that the ST segment is abolished. This is illustrated in Fig. 67.

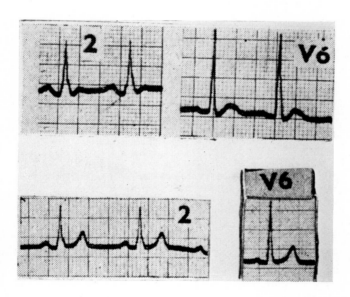

Fig. 67. *Upper tracing:* Hypercalcaemia. Note absent ST segment and short QT interval.

Lower tracing: Normal.

Hypocalcaemia. A low serum calcium may be found in hypoparathyroidism, uraemia, after hyperventilation, vomiting and massive transfusion of citrated blood. The QT interval is prolonged but this is mainly due to lengthening of the ST segment. This is

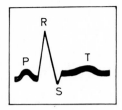

PROLONGED Q-T

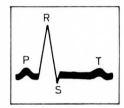

PROLONGED Q-T

FIG. 68. *Upper tracing:* Hypokalaemia (QT prolongation due to a low broad T wave).
   Lower tracing: Hypocalcaemia (QT prolongation due to a lengthened ST segment).

illustrated diagrammatically in Fig. 68 and is compared with the prolonged QT interval associated with hypokalaemia.

CARDIAC DRUGS

DIGITALIS

This is the 'great imitator' and is to the ECG what syphilis has been to medicine. Digitalis in therapeutic dosage most commonly produces changes in the ST segment and the T wave. These changes are as follows:—

(1) Depression of the ST segment in those leads in which the main deflection of the QRS is upright. The shape of the ST segment is distinctive and appears as a straight line running obliquely downward (the mirror image of a correction mark: $\sqrt{}$) or saucer-shaped with the concavity upwards (Fig. 69).

(2) Decrease in amplitude or even inversion of the T wave.

(3) Shortening of the QT interval.

Overdigitalization may produce various degrees of AV block, ventricular extrasystoles, often with coupled rhythm (pulsus bigeminus), nodal rhythm, atrial fibrillation, atrial tachycardia, ventricular tachycardia and, rarely, ventricular fibrillation.

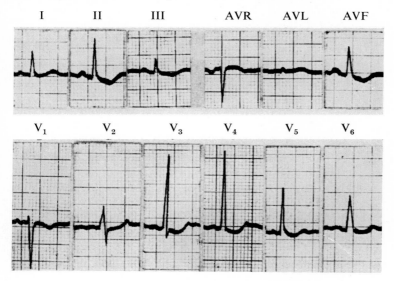

FIG. 69. Digitalis effect.

QUINIDINE

ECG changes associated with therapeutic doses of quinidine are:—

(1) Prolongation of the QT interval.

(2) Decrease in the amplitude or even inversion of the T wave, and

(3) ST segment depression.

Excessive amounts of quinidine may produce various types of conduction disturbances, AV block, prolongation of the QRS interval, ventricular fibrillation or cardiac standstill.

PROCAINE AMIDE

This drug should be administered intravenously slowly under ECG control until either the arrhythmia for which it is being used is controlled or signs of drug toxicity, such as ventricular extra-systoles, or a 50 per cent widening of the QRS complexes occur.

LIGNOCAINE

The use of this drug has been advocated for the treatment of ventricular arrhythmias following by-pass procedures (Weiss 1960). It should be administered in the same way as procaine amide and with the same precautions.

ISOPRENALINE

This drug stimulates the myocardium and increases the heart rate and stroke volume. It reduces peripheral vascular resistance, dilates the bronchial tree and does not cause potassium release from the liver. It is the drug of choice in the treatment of complete heart block occurring during open cardiac surgery and in the treatment of 'slow' ventricular fibrillation following elective cardiac arrest.

CHAPTER V

THE ELECTROCARDIOGRAM DURING ANAESTHESIA AND SURGERY

Within the operating theatre the ECG differs in two important aspects from one recorded in the out-patient clinic or in the ward. The first of these is the greater opportunity for the introduction of artefacts, and the second is the rapidly changing pattern of the recorded signal due to the effects of anaesthesia and surgery.

During anaesthesia and surgery conditions are frequently changing; there are alterations in the concentration of the anaesthetic agents administered, manoeuvres such as intubation, alterations in posture, respiration, temperature, blood pressure and pulse rate. Again pressor and cardiac drugs may be injected intravenously and electrolyte imbalance may be induced. Moreover, mechanical and physiological changes associated with the operation itself and massive blood transfusion may all alter the ECG pattern. To convey significant information, changes in the ECG pattern must be interpreted in the light of the stimulus producing them.

ARTEFACTS PECULIAR TO ELECTROCARDIOGRAPHY IN THE OPERATING THEATRE

AC INTERFERENCE OR 'HUM'

This may be produced by endoscopes *in situ*, e.g. bronchoscopes and cystoscopes when using mains reduction; by inadequate earthing of the ECG; or by inadequate earthing of other electrical apparatus, e.g. an electric blanket in use on the operating table. Interference produced by 50-cycle AC is illustrated in Fig. 59.

DIATHERMY CURRENT

The high frequency vibrations of the diathermy current completely obliterate the cardiac potentials and such interference is illustrated in Fig. 70.

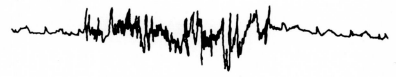

FIG. 70. Diathermy effect.

STATIC CHARGES

Large steel retractors, metal suckers, and scissors used during operation may induce static charges or may short circuit the cardiac potentials resulting in deflections which simulate extrasystoles (Fig. 71).

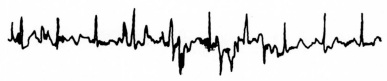

FIG. 71. Artefacts produced by retractors, metal suckers and scissors.

LOOSE ELECTRODES

Electrodes that are loose, or slip off, or are displaced by the operators beneath the towels may set up extraneous repetitive discharges which can simulate QRS complexes.

Patterns simulating the large Q waves and inverted T waves of myocardial infarction have been observed when one electrode was disconnected beneath the towels or a wire of the instrument cable was broken within the insulating sheath.

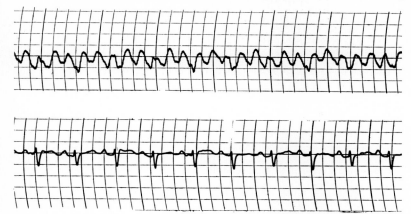

FIG. 72. *Upper tracing:* Sine wave artefact produced by pump oxygenator.
Lower tracing: The true ECG picture.

PUMP OXYGENATORS

A sine wave has been known to arise in a pump oxygenator and conducted to the patient through the arterial and venous channels and simulated a ventricular tachycardia as shown in Fig. 72.

INTRAVENTRICULAR STIMULATORS

These may be used in the treatment of heart block and produce the characteristic artefact illustrated in Fig. 73.

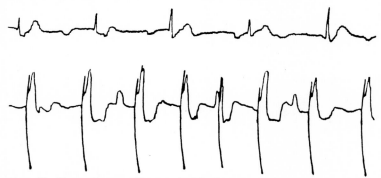

FIG. 73. *Upper tracing:* The true ECG picture.
Lower tracing: Artefact produced by an intraventricular stimulator (pacemaker).

MUSCLE FASCICULATION

This may follow an injection of suxamethonium or be associated with shivering during the induction of hypothermia or during the subsequent rewarming. It may simulate fibrillary and ectopic atrial contractions, which completely obscure the P waves, and is illustrated in Fig. 54.

DIAPHRAGMATIC CONTRACTIONS

These may be produced during periods of hiccough and during periods of tachypnoea associated with trichlorethylene or halothane anaesthesia and cause deflections which may resemble atrial ectopic beats (Fig. 74).

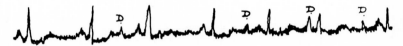

FIG. 74. Deflections produced by diaphragmatic contractions (D).

There is no single technique by which artefact can be recognized and eliminated. Very low or very high voltage in the recorded signal and abnormal wave forms different from the patient's pre-operative tracing should cause the anaesthetist to suspect artefact.

ECG CHANGES ASSOCIATED WITH INTUBATION, ENDOTRACHEAL SUCTION AND EXTUBATION

These are routine manoeuvres which usually are carried out without incident, but on occasion they have been associated with significant changes in the ECG pattern including cardiac arrest (Waters & Gillespie 1944; Nosworthy 1948; Gillespie 1948; Smith & Nolan 1950; Scurr 1950; Dale 1952; Fleming *et al* 1960; Bush *et al* 1962).

Many papers have been written on the ECG changes associated with these manoeuvres (Reid & Brace 1940; Burnstein *et al* 1950b, 1951; Peters *et al* 1951; Converse *et al* 1952; Fisher & Winsor 1952; Arcuri *et al* 1953; Rosner *et al* 1953; Stephen *et al* 1953;

Phillips 1954; Denson & Joseph 1954; Horton 1955; Jacoby *et al* 1955; Dance *et al* 1956; Rollason & Hough 1957b; Noble & Derrick 1959; Johnstone & Nisbet 1961). The changes most frequently observed included tachycardia, bradycardia, atrial, nodal and ventricular extrasystoles, atrial fibrillation, nodal rhythm, heart block, decrease in the height of the T wave and depression of the ST segment.

In the author's view, significant ECG changes during intubation, endotracheal suction or extubation are extremely rare in the absence of hypoxia, electrolyte imbalance or CO_2 retention.

It would however, appear that reflex cardiac arrest is more likely to occur during intubation in the severely burned patient (Fleming *et al* 1960; Bush *et al* 1962), but here toxaemia and electrolyte imbalance are probably predisposing factors.

Endoscopy, e.g. laryngoscopy, bronchoscopy and oesophagoscopy, like endotracheal intubation, often produces a marked pressor response (King *et al* 1951; Rollason & Hough 1957b). This will be referred to again under minor operative procedures.

ECG CHANGES ASSOCIATED WITH POSTURE AND CONTROLLED RESPIRATION

Changing the patient's posture, e.g. into the lateral or Trendelenburg positions may result in axis deviation. The employment of controlled respiration with deep inflation made possible by complete curarization or deep anaesthesia may also result in axis deviation and this is illustrated in Fig. 75.

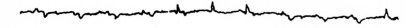

FIG. 75. Changes in electrical axis produced by controlled respiration.

Controlled respiration may, in addition, produce a sinus arrhythmia.

Certain types of surgery, particularly thoracotomy, may also produce both axis deviation and rotation of the heart.

ECG CHANGES DURING OCULAR SURGERY

Kirsch *et al* (1957) considered the oculocardiac reflex (Aschner 1908) to be more sensitive than the pulmocardiac reflex and found digital pressure on the globe, manipulation of the extra-ocular muscles and direct pressure on the tissue remaining in the apex of the orbit after enucleation could produce nodal rhythm, brady-cardia and transient cardiac arrest. These changes occurred under both local and general anaesthesia, but appeared to be abolished by a retrobulbar block. Bosomworth *et al* (1958) however, found retrobulbar block unsatisfactory but that Atropine was effective when given i.v. just prior to the commencement of surgery.

Other cases of cardiac arrest following traction to the extrinsic muscles of the eye have been reported (Sorbison & Gilmore 1956; Mallinson & Coombes 1960), and Deacock & Oxer (1962) recom-mended the use of gallamine for its vagal blocking activity during anaesthesia for procedures involving traction on the eye muscles.

ECG CHANGES DURING MINOR OPERATIVE PROCEDURES

ENDOSCOPY

The marked pressor response which can follow this procedure may place a considerable strain on a diseased heart, particularly if it is associated with anoxia and CO_2 retention. Under these circum-stances, the ECG pattern may reveal an arrhythmia, and/or changes in the ST segment and T wave suggesting myocardial anoxia, and on occasion, left ventricular 'strain'. Such changes would indicate the need to terminate the procedure and to ensure adequate oxygenation and ventilation of the patient. A ganglion blocking drug can prevent this response (Rollason & Hough 1957b), but may also produce hypotension. It may, however, be necessary to use one to prevent the massive autonomic response which can occur in paraplegics with cord lesions above the level of D6 during such procedures as cystoscopy and sigmoidoscopy.

CARDIAC CATHETERIZATION

During this procedure atrial and ventricular extrasystoles are common. If a dangerous arrhythmia, such as multifocal ventricular extrasystoles, develops, the catheter should be immediately withdrawn until the tip lies outside the heart, and the patient should be ventilated with pure oxygen, even though the blood gases at that stage have not been estimated. When pulmonary valvular stenosis has been diagnosed and cardiac catheterization is carried out on a patient with unsuspected Ebstein's malformation of the tricuspid valve, it may precipitate a fatal arrhythmia.

LEFT ATRIAL PUNCTURE

This is carried out through the chest wall and should be conducted under continuous ECG control, as it may be complicated by ventricular fibrillation. The ventricular fibrillation may be preceded by sinus arrest, idioventricular rhythm and broad QRS complexes, and if the procedure is rapidly terminated at this stage, a cardiac arrest may be avoided.

CORONARY ANGIOGRAPHY

This should also be conducted under continuous ECG control, particularly when hypotension is employed during the injection of the contrast medium. The systemic blood pressure can quickly be reduced by up to 50 per cent by inflation of the lungs with a constant pressure of 40 cm water during suxamethonium apnoea (Malmström *et al* 1960). When, however, abnormalities due to depressed conduction or ST deviation develop and are not obviously due to an anoxia which can be quickly remedied the investigation should be abandoned.

Some patients undergoing this procedure may have a high pulmonary vascular resistance and equally balanced left to right and right to left shunting and under these circumstances the institution of controlled ventilation may result in a sudden fall of arterial oxygen saturation with bradycardia and ECG changes indicative of myocardial ischaemia.

7

ECG CHANGES DURING CARDIAC SURGERY

Here the use of precordial leads is precluded and the anaesthetist must rely on the more remote limb leads. He has, however, the advantage of being able to observe the heart directly.

ST AND T WAVE CHANGES

Exposure of the surface of the heart to the drying action of the air and operating theatre lights, irritation of the myocardium by

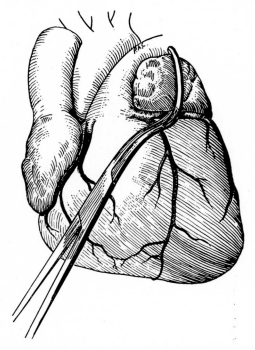

FIG. 76. (A) Clamp on the left atrial appendage involving the left coronary artery (B) ECG changes resulting from this.

irrigating fluids, retraction, and the administration of drugs, such as digitalis, have all been observed to produce ST segment and T wave changes without any evidence of hypoxia or obvious alteration in the patient's clinical condition. The non-specific nature of

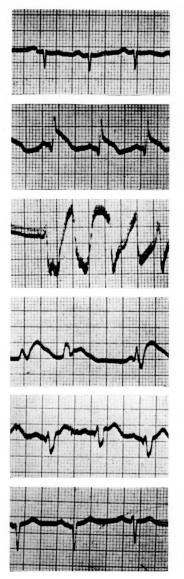

1. Tracing taken just prior to opening the thoracic cavity.

2. After occluding clamp applied. Note acute injury pattern simulating anterior myocardial infarction.

3. Ventricular fibrillation followed.

4. Position of occluding clamp was shifted and ventricular fibrillation ceased.

5. Temporary right B B B during closure of the atrial appendage.

6. During closure of the thoracic cavity the E C G returned essentially to normal and remained so.

Lead I taken in all tracings.

FIG. 76 (B).

these ST and T wave changes makes them a less reliable guide to myocardial oxygenation in the operating theatre than in the ward or consulting room. It is accordingly important to estimate myocardial oxygenation clinically by observing the colour of the heart and mucous membranes with a good light and against a white background.

When, however, ST segment and T wave changes are associated with myocardial anoxia, they are of the utmost importance and should be heeded without delay. If the hypoxia is due to respiratory obstruction or excessive hypotension, these must be remedied, forthwith. If due to interference with the blood supply to a portion of the myocardium, as for example, during a mitral valvotomy, when the posterior descending coronary artery may be occluded by pressure, the surgeon must be requested to remove his finger or valvulotome for a while. On the other hand, the changes may be due to the clamp on the left atrial appendage involving the left coronary artery (Fig. 76A, B). If the ST and T changes appear just after the placement of an intracardiac suture, a coronary artery branch may have been occluded and the suture should be removed.

A pericarditis pattern may be caused by the irritation of the subepicardial layer of muscle produced by 5 per cent trichloracetic acid and coarsely powdered asbestos applied to the epicardium in the Beck operation for the surgical treatment of myocardial ischaemia secondary to coronary artery disease. If left bundle branch block develops during this operation it is reputed to presage ventricular fibrillation and surgery should be terminated (Antonius *et al* 1956).

ARRYTHMIAS

(1) EXTRASYSTOLES

Different types of premature beat, atrial, nodal and ventricular are frequent during the surgical procedure, e.g. dislocation of the heart out of the pericardium during the Beck operation and during cardiotomy in cases of atrial and ventricular septal defect, valvular pulmonary stenosis and the Tetralogy of Fallot.

(2) PAROXYSMAL TACHYCARDIA

Should supraventricular tachycardia develop, e.g. during the Beck operation, and if the patient has received no previous digitalis, 0·5 mg digoxin well diluted, can safely be given slowly by IV injection and repeated once if necessary after half an hour.

(3) ATRIAL FIBRILLATION

Short bouts of this may also be observed.

(4) AV BLOCK

Generally the cause for this is immediately apparent, as in its occurrence with the placement of a suture in the heart which has interrupted impulse conduction within the bundle of His, or one of its branches. Removal of the offending suture usually results in the return of a normal conduction pattern.

Transient AV block or intraventricular block (idioventricular rhythm) frequently follows mitral valvotomy, but the normal conduction pattern returns soon after the surgeon's finger or valvulotome is removed from the heart.

If complete heart block develops during an open heart procedure, it may be necessary to treat it by suturing electrodes to the ventricular epicardium and connecting them to a pacemaker. External and internal cardiac pacemakers have been developed which give painless and effective control of the heart rate (Abrams et al 1960; Portal et al 1962; Glass et al 1963).

Although Ross (1962) has advocated the use of ether for patients with complete heart block halothane skilfully administered appears to be quite satisfactory in the presence of adequate pacing and avoids the explosive hazard (Howat 1963).

(5) VENTRICULAR FIBRILLATION

This is not an infrequent accompaniment of cardiac surgery and anaesthesia and will be discussed under ECG changes associated with special techniques.

ECG CHANGES ASSOCIATED WITH
SPECIAL TECHNIQUES

INDUCED HYPOTENSION

The arguments for and against induced hypotension have continued unabated since its introduction by Gardner in 1946. Many, however, feel that in skilled hands it carries no great risk, provided tachycardia is avoided, vasodilatation is ensured and a constant blood volume is maintained (Rollason 1953). Ganglionic blocking drugs per se do not appear to produce significant changes in the ECG and many ECG studies have been conducted during hypotensive anaesthesia produced by ganglionic blockade, either by methonium-like compounds or by spinal or epidural analgesia. Some workers (Enderby 1951; James *et al* 1953; Mandow *et al* 1954; Stirling 1955) producing sympathetic blockade with methonium compounds and others (Lynn *et al* 1952) employing spinal blockade found no significant ECG changes during the period of induced hypotension. Other investigators, however, (Davison 1951; Longtin 1952, 1954; Camerini *et al* 1952, 1958; Swerdlow & Wade 1953; Wyman 1953; Wenger *et al* 1953; Van Bergen *et al* 1954; Haid 1954; Gordon & Ladenheim 1955; Mazzia *et al* 1956; Rollason & Cumming 1956) have reported significant ECG changes in a proportion of cases, during induced hypotension produced by ganglion blocking drugs. Should the BP be allowed to fall too low, reduction in the height of the P wave, nodal rhythm, and ST segment and T wave changes appear (Fig. 77, 78). Occasionally the pattern improves as the pressure falls (Fig. 79). ST segment depression greater than 1 mm which persists and a flattening or inversion of the T wave are indications for raising the BP. The incidence of the ECG changes is significantly higher and their magnitude greater when the hypotension is associated with tachycardia (Rollason & Hough 1959, 1960b. & c). This is more likely to be the case if ganglion blocking drugs or gallamine are employed in the technique (Fig. 80). Hypotension produced by spinal analgesia or halothane and oxygen alone is associated with a slow pulse rate. The halothane technique has been routinely employed by the author since 1957, without any untoward sequelae which could be definitely related to the method provided adequate oxygenation and ventilation is ensured throughout, and the BP is not permitted to fall below 60 mm Hg in the normotensive or 80 mm in the case of patients with marked systolic hypertension. Respiration is controlled throughout (Rollason 1960, Murtagh 1960). Transient ST and T wave changes may however occur if the rate of fall is precipitous (Rollason *et al* 1963).

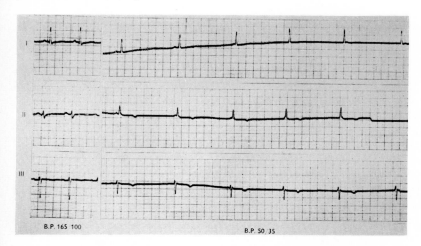

Fig. 77. Transitions from sinus to superior nodal, nodal and inferior nodal rhythm during the hypotensive phase. T wave flattening and inversion are also seen.

Should bradycardia become extreme, i.e. if the pulse rate falls below 40 beats per minute, when employing this technique, a normal rate can be restored by the intravenous injection of atropine which also results in a rise in BP.

In order to correct the tachycardia sometimes associated with ganglion blocking drugs, hydergine (Rollason & Hough 1959, 1960a), procaine amide (Mason & Pelmore 1953; Aserman 1953) and guanethidine (Holloway *et al* 1961) have been used. Hydergine and guanethidine in the dosage used do not appear *per se* to produce significant changes in the ECG, but procaine amide on the other hand, depresses conduction and should be stopped if ventric-

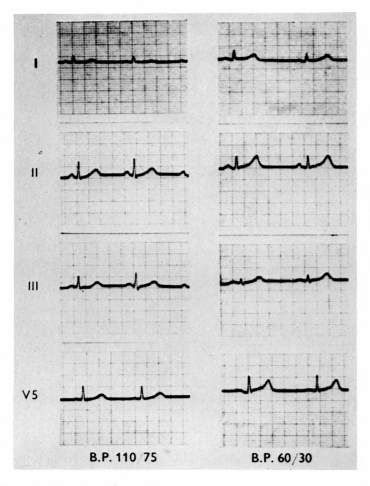

FIG. 78. Elevation of the ST segment and increase in the height of the T wave during the hypotensive phase.

ular extrasystoles appear or if the QRS interval increases by 50 per cent, otherwise asystole or ventricular fibrillation may ensue. These cardiotoxic effects are, however, reputed to be reversed in dogs by the use of 4 m eq/Kg of molar sodium lactate (Bellet *et al* 1959).

Induced hypotension and the foetus

Ebner *et al* (1960) studied the effect of post-spinal hypotension on the foetal ECG and found that foetal bradycardia developed when the maternal systolic BP dropped to 60 mm Hg for a period longer than 4 minutes. Smyth (1962), however, is of the opinion that the appearance of extrasystoles in the foetal ECG constitutes the first sign of anoxia.

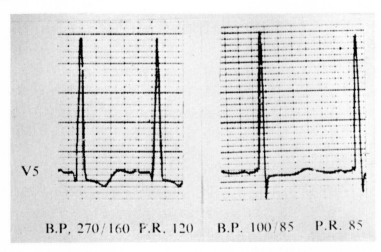

B.P. 270/160 F.R. 120   B.P. 100/85   P.R. 85

FIG. 79. Disappearance of left ventricular 'strain' pattern during the hypotensive phase in a case of malignant hypertension. The improved pattern is probably due to a relatively greater reduction in cardiac work than coronary flow. Slowing of the P.R. may also be a factor.

INDUCED HYPOTHERMIA

When dogs are cooled so that their rectal temperature falls below 25°C, the ECG shows a current of injury (Osborn 1953). This consists of a displacement of the junction of the QRS complex and the ST segment, the so-called J deflection. This is illustrated in Fig. 81.

The J deflection is not infrequently seen during routine hypothermia in man, and appears to have no special significance. It is certainly valueless as a warning of ventricular fibrillation (Emslie Smith *et al* 1959).

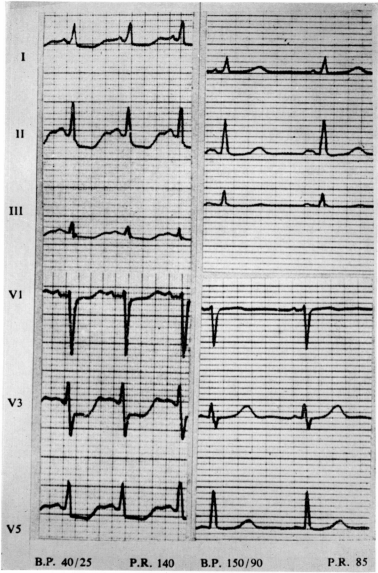

B.P. 40/25 P.R. 140 B.P. 150/90 P.R. 85

FIG. 80. *Tracings on the left:* Illustrate the gross ST depression. which can be associated with a combination of tachycardia and hypotension.

Tracings on the right: Illustrate that these changes are reversible when the BP is raised and the PR slowed.

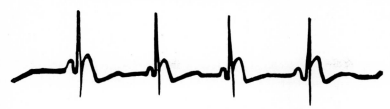

FIG. 81. The Osborn wave.

In man, sinus bradycardia, together with a reduction in the height of the P wave or nodal rhythm, are frequent accompaniments of cooling in the absence of shivering. It is due to depression of the SA node and conduction through the bundle of His. Cardiac systole takes up a greater than normal fraction of the cycle, and below 30°C (86°F) these conduction changes are manifested by a prolonged PR interval, widening of the QRS complex and lengthening of the ST interval. These are illustrated in Fig. 82. Deviations

9 40
98.4°F M.H.

11·45
85°F M·H.

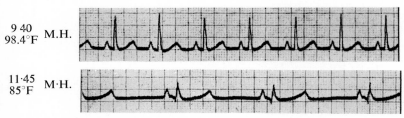

FIG. 82. *Upper tracing* is normal.
   Lower tracing shows prolongation of the PR, QRS and ST intervals during induced hypothermia.

of the ST segment, changes in the amplitude and direction of the T wave and atrial fibrillation are not infrequently seen during hypothermia in clinical practice. Extrasystoles and runs of ventricular tachycardia may end in ventricular fibrillation at temperatures below 28°C (82·4°F). It should, however, be stressed that ventricular fibrillation in hypothermia can occur without any previous changes in the ECG pattern. It is of interest to note that quinidine sulphate has been shown to lower the incidence of ventricular fibrillation during induced hypothermia in dogs (Currie *et al* 1962).

Multifocal ventricular extrasystoles or ventricular tachycardia

have been consistently observed during hypothermia following
removal of the clamps used for inflow occlusion during the operation for pulmonary valvotomy and for the repair of atrial septal
defects (Cannard *et al* 1960). The heart is extremely irritable immediately following restoration of the circulation and remains so for
several minutes (Fig. 83). All mechanical stimulation should be

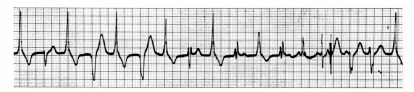

FIG. 83. Myocardial irritability immediately following restoration of
the circulation.

avoided following release of the occluding clamps until the ECG
shows less myocardial irritability as indicated by disappearance of
the extrasystoles and return to the control pattern.

PROFOUND HYPOTHERMIA

When hypothermia is used by itself, the customary limit of cooling
is 28–30°C (82·4–86°F). At this level of temperature, circulatory
arrest and open heart surgery is possible for 8–10 minutes only.

In 'profound' hypothermia, the patient is cooled to 14°C (57·2°F)
which permits circulatory arrest for a period of up to 52 minutes
(Benazon 1960). In this technique, the ECG undergoes changes
characteristic of cooling, bradycardia being followed by varying
degrees of heart block, culminating in ventricular fibrillation.
Atrial fibrillation is not as a rule observed. Occasionally, the atria
continue to beat at a slow rate in the presence of ventricular
fibrillation.

The ECG during ventricular fibrillation often shows a characteristic wave form of groups of complexes (Fig. 84). When this
pattern has become well established, the ECG carries a good prog-
nosis as defibrillation often occurs spontaneously on rewarming.

During the period of circulatory arrest there is a state of suspended animation, cardiac and respiratory functions are in abeyance and the ECG unless the heart is fibrillating is inactive.

During rewarming, when the pharyngeal temperature reaches 30–34°C (86–93·2°F) a single electric shock, or simply manual stimulation, is usually sufficient to restore regular rhythm in the fibrillating heart. Often fibrillation is not seen at any time during the operation, particularly in young children. On the other hand, sinus rhythm can be restored after prolonged fibrillation, provided the heart is warm, well oxygenated and not overdistended.

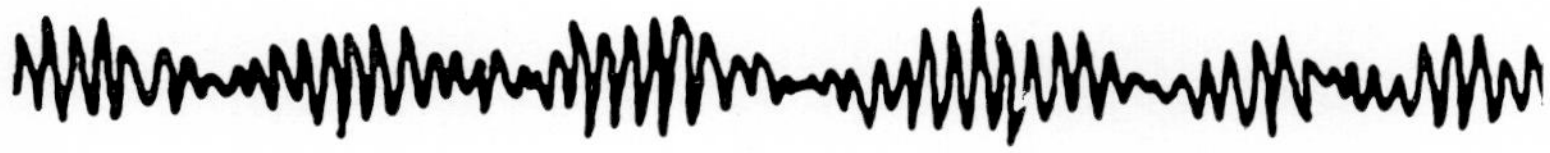

FIG. 84. Ventricular fibrillation pattern during profound hypothermia illustrating groups of complexes.

EXTRACORPOREAL CIRCULATION AND ELECTIVE CARDIAC ARREST

This may be used in association with or without hypothermia. The ECG is particularly valuable when the heart cannot be directly observed, in indicating changes in heart rate and in portraying arrhythmias, particularly complete heart block which indicates the need for a large intravenous dose of atropine (1–2 mg), or isoprenaline (0·5–1·0 mg). If these are not effective, it may be necessary to resort to the artificial pacemaker, both during the operation and in the post-operative period.

The onset of supraventricular tachycardia with the accompanying signs of myocardial failure, may be an indication for immediate digitalization. If the tachycardia and hypotension fail to respond, then a small dose of neostigmine sulphate (0·5–1·0 mg) should be tried.

For ventricular arrhythmias after by-pass, intravenous 2 per cent lignocaine may be given in a dose of 1 mg per kg body-weight, every 10 minutes (Weiss 1960; Weiss & Bailey 1960).

When direct coronary perfusion is employed, its adequacy can be determined by the ECG. After temporary elective cardiac arrest with potassium chloride, or acetylcholine, special coronary perfusion cannulae are placed in the coronary ostia. Coronary perfusion is thus instituted by an auxiliary pump drawing blood from the arterial end of the oxygenator. The coronary perfusion rate is increased until the myocardium is pink and the ECG resembles the pre by-pass pattern. Should air inadvertently gain access into the coronoary vessels, ischaemic ECG changes will be observed.

The ECG can be most useful in determining the diagnosis and the result of treatment of arrhythmias, especially subsequent to elective cardiac arrest.

During the onset of elective cardiac arrest, the ECG shows bradycardia, absence of atrial activity and broadening of the QRS component, i.e. the picture of the 'dying heart'. Ventricular tachycardia and ventricular fibrillation may occur due to an insufficient or too slow injection of the arresting agent. During arrest the heart is in diastole and overfilling must be prevented by early ventriculotomy.

During recovery the ventriculotomy should not be closed until vigorous heart action has been established. This may be preceded by varying grades of heart block, ventricular tachycardia or ventricular fibrillation necessitating electrical defibrillation.

Before attempting defibrillation, efforts should be made to improve perfusion and oxygenation of the myocardium. During electrical defibrillation, a considerable decrease in pO_2 in the arterial end of the oxygenator is noted. This occurs at a time when adequate oxygenation is of prime importance, i.e. during defibrillation. The massive contractions of skeletal muscle which occur with electric shock increase the consumption of oxygen and may mobilize quantities of grossly desaturated blood pooled in the peripheral areas of the body. This results in a flooding of this grossly desaturated venous blood into the oxygenator. The administration of a paralysing dose of relaxant into the oxygenator prior to defibrillation prevents this drop in pO_2 as well as the accidental dislodgement of ECG electrodes or one of the numerous cannulae connected to the patient.

During electrical defibrillation, the ECG should be switched off to prevent damage to the instrument. Saline applied to the heart can cause ST segment depression and T wave inversion (Milstein 1961), and it has been recommended that mammalian Ringer's solution should be used on the gauze or lint on the defibrillator electrodes (Shepherd 1961).

The diagnosis of 'slow' ventricular fibrillation after elective cardiac arrest cannot, however, be made with the ECG, but is made by direct observation of the heart (Mendelsohn et al 1960). The ventricles present a worm-like flaccid appearance. Electrical defibrillation is usually impossible, but isoprenaline has proved an effective defibrillating agent.

ECG CHANGES ASSOCIATED WITH TRANSFUSIONS OF BLOOD AND PLASMA

Some cases of cardiac arrest encountered during anaesthesia appear to be due to massive blood transfusion or to the transfusion of concentrated or fresh frozen plasma and the anaesthetist when supervising one of these transfusions should have the benefit of continuous ECG control. The critical factor suggested is the ratio of potassium to calcium in the venous return to the heart; should this ratio become excessively large, as may be found in blood over three or four days old, cardiac arrest may follow (Le Veen et al 1960; Gain 1962; Bunker et al 1962). For this reason, the addition of 10 per cent calcium gluconate or 10 per cent calcium chloride (which ionizes more rapidly) to the citrated blood has been advised (Ludbrook & Wynn 1958; Marshall 1962), but the value of this practice would appear to be open to question, for it has been shown that in patients who received calcium salts during high rates of blood administration had a higher mortality rate than patients not receiving calcium (Howland et al 1960; Boyan & Howland 1962). Moreover, it has been shown in humans that the intravenous administration of 2·7 g calcium chloride in 3 minutes can cause nodal rhythm, heart block and ventricular extrasystoles (Clarke 1941). Should, however, tall tented T waves and prolonged QT intervals develop during the transfusion of blood or plasma, particularly in small children whose reservoir of tissue fluid in relation to their blood volume is small, it would appear advisable to inject 10 per cent calcium gluconate or chloride slowly intravenously *pari passu* with the blood or plasma until the ECG changes are reversed. Should a cardiac stimulant be indicated, adrenaline should be avoided as it releases potassium from the liver. Isoprenaline, which does not have this action and is a more effective stimulant should be the drug of choice in these circumstances.

As selective cooling of the heart can produce arrest, it would seem advisable to pass an appropriate length of the transfusion tubing conducting the refrigerated blood to the patient, through a water bath at 37°C (98·4°F) (Boyan & Howland 1961), and when practicable to monitor the central venous pressure, as a rise in the latter may indicate a failure of cardiac contractability or over-loading of the circulation before ECG changes, such as a right ventricular 'strain' pattern, are manifest.

As hypothermia to 28°–29°C (82·4–84·2°F) reduces the rate of metabolic destruction of citrate (Krebs cycle) by 30–40 per cent, it would appear wise when massive transfusion is anticipated, to avoid citrated blood and to use either heparinized blood or blood treated with ethylene-diamine-tetra-acetic acid (EDTA) and to guard against excessive selective cooling of the heart except in cases undergoing open cardiac surgery.

The development of sudden gross ischaemic ECG changes should lead the anaesthetist to suspect air embolism, but this hazard should be appreciated and prevented as it should also be in the case of patients being operated on in the sitting position.

The need for massive transfusion on the one hand must be weighted against the danger of circulatory overloading and pulmonary oedema on the other, particularly in chest injuries and during a pneumonectomy when the ECG should be observed for evidence of right heart 'strain'.

ECG changes may on occasion be associated with transfusions other than those of blood and plasma. Dehydration therapy with 30 per cent urea for instance may result in the appearance of elevated ST segments and inverted T waves.

CHAPTER VI

ELECTROCARDIOGRAPHIC EQUIPMENT SUITABLE FOR USE BY THE ANAESTHETIST

It is difficult to make any recommendations for the type of equipment suitable for this use, as both the purpose and the financial resources of different anaesthetists vary. It is possible for research to be undertaken in a specialist unit at a teaching centre with every facility, or in a busy peripheral general hospital with practically no resources save the enthusiasm of the anaesthetist. Routine ECGs may be taken on special equipment belonging to the operating theatre or on equipment borrowed from the cardiological unit of the hospital. In some instances, a skilled ECG technician may be available but in many cases the anaesthetist will have to operate the machine himself. It seems best, therefore, to discuss ECG machines in general and then to consider what features are particularly desirable for routine and research use.

ELECTROCARDIOGRAPHIC MACHINES

It is not proposed to give a detailed account of the design of ECG machines, as this would involve an unnecessary incursion into the field of electronics. An attempt will be made to describe the underlying principles and to explain the features which make certain types of machines particularly suitable for use in the theatre.

The purpose of an ECG machine is to detect the changes of potential produced by the heart between two electrodes placed at suitable positions on the patient, and to make these changes visible to the observer. The potential to be detected is quite small, of the order of 1 mV, and the changes in potential occur rapidly (the QRS complex only lasts from 0·05 to 0·10 second) and is super-imposed on the skin current which is DC potential, which may be as great as 20 mV, and varies slowly with time. The machine must separate the potential due to the heart from the skin current, amplify it and then record the result in either a permanent or a temporary form. In the earliest types of machine, amplification was avoided by using an exceptionally sensitive detector—usually a string galvanometer; unfortunately, the high sensitivity of the detector made the instrument both fragile and very sensitive to external vibrations. The string galvanometer type of detector is not really suitable for portable instruments and it is rapidly passing out of use, even for permanent installations. Enthoven's original string galvanometer consisted of an exceedingly fine wire, such as silver coated glass, suspended between the poles of an electromagnet; when a current passed through the fibre, the latter was deflected towards one pole or the other, according to the direction of the current. By suitable magnification and illumination, the movements of the shadow of this string could be recorded on a moving photographic film.

It is from this galvanometer that the modern electrocardiograph has evolved.

The design of the electronic circuit of a modern instrument will not be discussed. The important point is that the circuit requires a source of electric power—either the AC mains or a battery. The introduction of transistors in place of thermionic valves resulted in a reduction of both size and power consumption.

It is the recorder which is the aspect of greatest significance to the anaesthetist. If it is to follow faithfully the shape of the potential between the electrodes, it must be capable of travelling several centimetres in 0·01 second and be capable of making rapid changes in direction without lag. Mathematicians have shown that it is possible to estimate the way in which a recorder will follow a complicated voltage pattern from the way in which it responds to simple sine waves of different frequencies. To follow the potential wave from the heart, the recorder should have a flat response from about 1 c/s up to about 500 c/s. In a practical recorder this requirement has also to be related to the ease with which the record can be read. Four main types of recorder can be distinguished, (1) photographic, (2) stylus, (3) jet and (4) cathode ray oscillograph.

The earliest type of recorder was the photographic and this was used on the early string galvanometer electrocardiographic machines. It has the great advantage that moving parts are light in weight and that the distance they move is magnified by the light beam; consequently, it is not difficult to produce a recorder which has the required frequency response. The big disadvantage of this type of recorder is that the record is not immediately available and that a dark-room is needed to develop the record. It is now possible to produce a special type of photographic recorder using ultraviolet light and to make the record immediately available; such a recorder is more complex than the normal type and also more expensive.

The earliest types of 'direct writer', i.e. machines which provide a visible permanent record immediately employed a stylus recording directly on paper. This means that the pen has to travel several centimetres over paper and it is very difficult to maintain a satisfactory response to the higher frequencies; consequently, the finer details of the ECG are lost and the record is inferior to that produced by a photographic recorder. With this type of recorder, there is a tendency for the record to be distorted, and for the time marker lines to be curved on the chart to compensate for this. The stylus may record on the paper in three different ways, (1) by the use of an ink reservoir (2) by a heated stylus recording on special paper or (3) by passing a current between the stylus and backing sheet through special paper. Both the latter methods may be dangerous in the operating theatre if an inflammable anaesthetic is being used and should be avoided.

An ingenious method of overcoming the poor high frequency response of the stylus direct writer is the use of a jet of ink in place of the conventional stylus (Fig. 85). This method has produced ECG machines with a very good frequency response with the advantage of also being real direct writers (Fig. 86). The main difficulty with this design is that the galvanometer unit is liable to

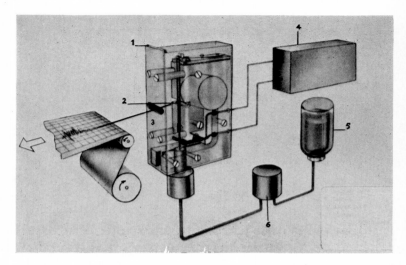

FIG. 85. The ink jet principle. (1) galvanometer casing (2) nozzle (3) jet of fluid (4) amplifier (5) writing fluid bottle (6) pump. A loop of wire is suspended in a magnetic field. Attached to this wire is a fine bore glass nozzle (2), weighing only a fraction of a milligram. When electric current is fed into the loop, it rotates, taking with it the nozzle. Writing fluid is supplied through a central capillary and during registration forced through the nozzle under high pressure (approximately 25 atmospheres) on the passing graph paper. The jet of fluid is only 0·01 mm in diameter and replaces the stylus arm used in conventional direct recorders.

trouble with the jet becoming blocked, or if the ink reservoir is allowed to get too low.

Another method of recording ECGs is only a transient one, as they are displayed on the screen of a cathode ray oscillograph with long afterglow. This makes it possible to see the ECG, but it soon fades away; it is usual to use this method to follow the behaviour of the heart over a long period and hence it has the name of 'monitor'. Most of the monitors at present produced are designed to be used in conjunction with an existing ECG machine, but there is now a simple self-contained monitor available—the Videograph —which is illustrated in Fig. 87. The great advantages of this method are that the picture on the screen is easier to see and no

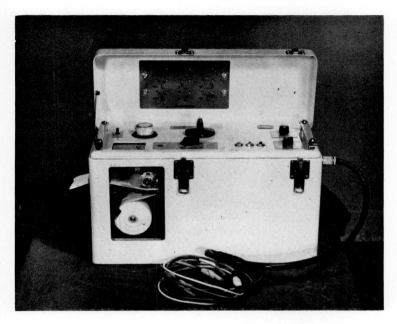

FIG. 86. The Mingograf 12 which incorporates the ink jet principle.

expensive paper is needed to record; during an operation of several hours duration, it would need several hundred metres of paper to keep a continuous record and this is difficult to study as well as expensive.

All recorders are made in either a single channel type or a type to record two or more ECGs simultaneously (multi-channel). Most of the multi-channel types can be adjusted to permit the recording of the output of other physiological parameters simultaneously with the ECG, e.g. the EEG and pressure measurements. It is of great value to be able to record simultaneously, as it permits the accurate correlation of the different parameters. The simultaneous recording of the standard leads is necessary if the orientation of the QRS voltage is to be studied (changes in a single lead may be due to only axis deviation which may not be very significant).

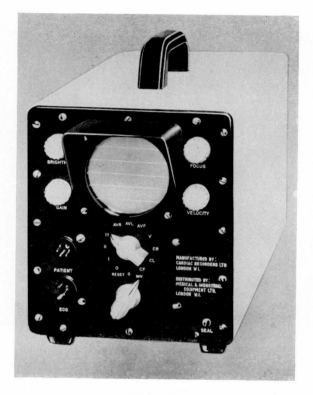

Fig. 87. The videograph.

ECG MACHINES FOR USE DURING
ROUTINE ANAESTHESIA

The reason for using an ECG machine during routine anaesthesia is to detect quickly changes in the condition of the patient's heart, so that immediate steps can be taken to prevent serious conditions developing. Ordinary photographic recording is unsuitable for this purpose, as it is necessary to develop the film before it yields its information; the choice is between direct writers and a monitor. It is too expensive to use a direct writer continuously throughout a routine procedure, and so the ideal instrument is a monitor. In practice, it is usual to link the monitor to a direct writer and this

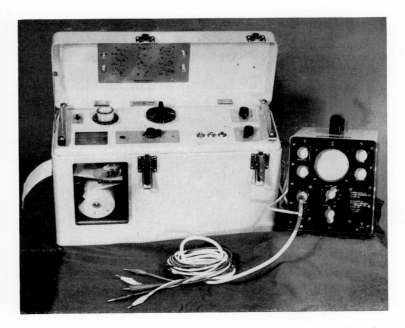

FIG. 88. Mingograf 12 linked to videograph. The selector control on the Mingograf is left at the lead I setting while the selector control on the Videograph is used to select serially the various lead positions and the tracings from these can be portrayed on both the scope and the direct writer or on the scope alone.

enables permanent records to be obtained when interesting changes are observed on the monitor (Fig. 88).

It is advisable to make arrangements with the theatre sister about the positioning of the machine and of the leads to the patient. Space is sometimes limited and by obtaining good co-operation it will be much easier to see that a position is found which will enable the anaesthetist to see the monitor easily and at the same time not interfere with the surgical team.

Some monitors have a floor stand but it is often more convenient to have the smaller type which can stand on a stool, table, top of a diathermy machine, etc.

ECG MACHINES FOR ANAESTHETIC RESEARCH

For research purposes, it is not usually necessary to analyse the record immediately and so the major disadvantage of photographic recording disappears and the very good record produced by this means is a real advantage. In research investigation, it is usually desirable to use a multi-channel recorder. Other variables of interest are EEG, arterial and central venous pressures, respiratory volume, etc. It is becoming standard practice to combine many of the instruments for recording these parameters into a single trolley, and it would be desirable to consider carefully whether such a trolley should not be purchased when planning a new research project. Most of these trolleys incorporate one or more oscilloscopes, so that it is possible to monitor the variables and to record when there is an indication that significant changes are occurring.

The use of a single trolley with the complete physiological recording equipment on it has the great advantage that it simplifies the setting up of equipment in the theatre and also reduces the floor area required. Research is always an activity which tends to conflict with the most efficient performance of routine surgery and all steps which reduce the interference will assist in obtaining the willing co-operation of the surgical team which is essential if good research is to be done. A single trolley makes it easier for the anaesthetist to undertake the recording himself and certainly makes it possible to only need a single research assistant. A trolley, incorporating ECG, EEG and a twin scope, used by the author is illustrated in Fig. 89.

A most essential aspect of any investigation is to ensure that the equipment is in good working order and has been carefully set up and standardized before the start of the operation. It is never easy to arrange to make an adequate number of observations and it is very disappointing when observations during a particular operation have to be abandoned due to the failure of the instrument, or the results discarded because it is clear that the instrument was not correctly standardized. The most satisfactory procedure is to have the same team on all occasions and to work with the same theatre staff and surgeon; adequate time must be allowed for both the preliminary check of the equipment and also for setting up and final calibration in the theatre. It may well take five or six occasions before the drill has been really well established and it will then be found that reproducible results can be obtained.

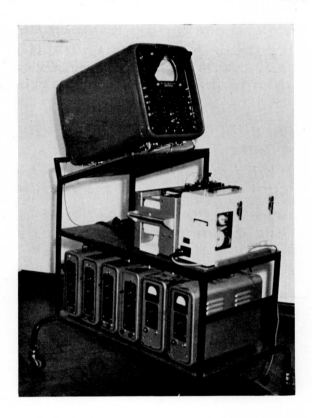

FIG. 89. ECG, EEG and twin scope mounted on a single trolley.

Research investigations can be done with quite simple equipment and any ECG machine available can be pressed into service. The previous suggestions have assumed that a research unit is being set up and that reasonable funds are available. Much of the published work on ECG changes during anaesthesia has been done on single channel direct writers.

ELECTRICAL INTERFERENCE

ECG practice is always much concerned about electrical interference; the record is frequently marred by the superposition of
electric potentials not produced by the heart. DC potentials are
eliminated by the same procedure as skin current but alternating
potentials cannot be. The usual source of interference is the AC
mains. AC interference is illustrated in Fig. 59. In an ECG
department it is possible to design the electric installations in such
a way that this is minimized but clearly in the operating theatre
cables carrying the AC mains must run in the vicinity of the operating table for the various items of theatre equipment. The leads
from the patient to the machine are always in the form of screened
cables and so the main source of interference is the AC potentials
induced in the patient. The effect of these can be very much reduced
by ensuring that there is a good contact between the patient and
the electrode. For this reason the screw-on needle types of electrode
are to be preferred. An extra earth lead connected externally in
series to all electrical apparatus in use in the theatre may also assist
in eliminating AC interference.

In the theatre, there is that gross source of interference — the
diathermy. When the diathermy machine is working, the ECG pattern either disappears completely or suffers from gross interference
(Fig. 70). There is virtually nothing that can be done to eliminate
this interference. The potentials induced can become so great that
damage may be done to some types of machine; it is possible to
arrange a circuit such that when the diathermy is in use it auto-
matically cuts out the ECG machine.

If severe interference is found to occur in a particular theatre, it
is often possible to reduce its effect by repositioning the ECG
machine and rearranging the various electric cables to the table. It
is not possible to suggest a systematic method of finding the best
position; trial and error is the only way.

ELECTRODES FOR ELECTROCARDIOGRAPHY

There is a considerable difference between the requirements for
electrodes in operating theatres and those for electrocardiography

carried out in the out-patient clinic or the ward. In a cardiological department, the patient only wears the electrodes for a few minutes and it is quite easy to adjust them should a poor contact develop. In the theatre, it is quite common for observations to extend over several hours and it is often quite impossible to adjust an electrode during surgery. The electrodes usually supplied by manufacturers are not always suitable for theatre use (it is common to find that even ECG departments prefer a different type of electrode). The requirements are (1) a good contact to reduce interference and

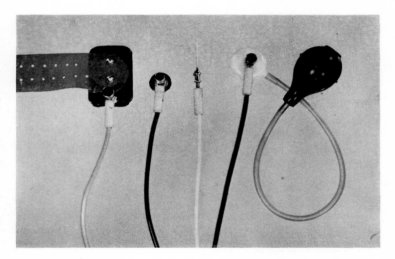

Fig. 90. Types of electrode. Left to right: Plate, disc, needle and suction electrodes.

improve the record and (2) a contact which will be satisfactory over a period of several hours.

Two types of electrode have been found suitable for this use, the needle and disc (button) electrodes (Fig. 90). The needle is probably the most satisfactory of all but it is clearly unsuitable when it is desired to make observations continuously during the induction of anaesthesia and during the recovery period. Using the disc electrode, electrode jelly and strapping on the back of the disc normally ensure an adequate contact for considerable periods.

The position of the electrodes for the standard leads may have to be varied along the limb to allow for the posture of the patient and the requirements of surgery. This is not important and substantially the same record will be obtained for any position along the limb.

Occasionally it may be necessary to have a lead and its electrode sterilized and placed *in situ* by the surgeon.

In order to ensure the accurate placement of chest electrodes in the taking of serial ECG tracings, a grid has been evolved by Kerwin *et al* (1960) and a calliper by Rose (1961).

EXTERNAL ELECTRIC STIMULATOR

In recent years, it has been found possible to treat ventricular standstill by the use of an external electric stimulator or 'artificial pacemaker'; as asystole may occur during anaesthesia and surgery, it is likely that the anaesthetist will be responsible for initiating treatment and supervising the patient during the period whilst treatment continues. It is usual to use an ECG monitor to supervise the patient and in order to prevent extended periods of personal supervision, the more recent instruments have an automatic device incorporated within them so that the ECG machine switches the stimulator off and on as required. A typical machine has been described by Leatham *et al* (1956) and Portal *et al* (1963) have stressed its value in cardiac resuscitation.

More recently, as a result of the development during open cardiac surgery of complete heart block, myocardial electrodes are sutured into the epicardium of the heart and connected to a pacemaker. It is important that the ECG should be adequately earthed for should this not be so, and the patient is at the same time earthed via the pacemaker electrodes sutured into the epicardium, it is possible for a current of ImA to pass directly through the heart which is very sensitive to electrical impulses and if a current of this magnitude passes for longer than 0·1 second, it may be sufficient to cause ventricular fibrillation (Noordijk *et al* 1961).

CHAPTER VII

THE VALUE AND LIMITATIONS OF THE ECG

The ECG provides the anaesthetist with a record of the heart rate, its rhythm, the site and number of the pacemakers, the efficiency of the conducting tissue and the position of the heart. It provides a means of recording fluctuations of autonomic tone produced by the various drugs used by him or his surgical and cardiological colleagues, and is a valuable index of the electrolyte balance of the blood. It is essentially a picture of the site of origin of the stimulus potential and the speed and direction in which it travels to initiate the myocardial contraction. As the conducting system and the myocardium derive their nutrient from a common blood supply, i.e. the coronary arteries, it seems reasonable to assume that any drugs or manoeuvres which produce electrocardiographic evidence of impairment of one may involve impairment of the other (Johnstone 1956). The ECG can be a valuable aid to the anaesthetist pre-operatively, during surgery and anaesthesia and in the post-operative period. The ECG changes, however, must be interpreted in the pre-operative period in conjunction with the clinical findings, in the theatre in conjunction with the events immediately preceding them, and in the post-operative period with the operation performed.

PRE-OPERATIVELY

The ECG is of particular value in elucidating the following conditions:

1. cardiomegaly

2. myocardial infarction (if recent elective surgery should be postponed for 3–6 months)

3. cardiac arrhythmia

4. pericarditis

5. systemic diseases affecting the myocardium

6. the effects of cardiac drugs, e.g. digitalis

7. electrolyte imbalance, e.g. hypokalaemia in diabetes mellitus and hyperkalaemia in uraemia

DURING ANAESTHESIA AND SURGERY

Here the ECG is valuable:

(1) In the evaluation of new agents, drugs and techniques.

(2) In the immediate detection of cardiac arrest and whether this is due to ventricular fibrillation or to asystole. A case of cardiac arrest occurring during an abdomino-perineal resection and its response to cardiac massage is illustrated in Fig. 91.

(3) As a continuous monitor portraying evidence of myocardial ischaemia, arrhythmia or electrolyte imbalance during

    (a) hypotensive anaesthesia

    (b) hypothermia

    (c) cardiac and vascular surgery

    (d) removal of a phaeochromocytoma and

    (e) any type of surgery in the poor risk case

The development of the following (i) gross ST segment and/or T wave changes, (ii) excessive widening of the QRS complex, with extrasystoles, and absent P waves (the 'dying heart'), (iii) multifocal ventricular extrasystoles, (iv) complete heart block, and (v) tall tented T waves with a prolonged QT interval, should all be viewed with concern and immediate remedial action taken.

The development of a right or left ventricular 'strain' pattern may constitute an indication for intravenous digitalization and a tachycardia above 160 or a bradycardia below 40 should not be allowed to persist.

POST-OPERATIVELY

The ECG may be of value as a continuous monitor in the recovery ward, but more particularly so in the intensive therapy unit. The prompt recognition of an arrhythmia and skilful treatment may well determine the success of the surgical procedure (Buckley & Jackson 1961).

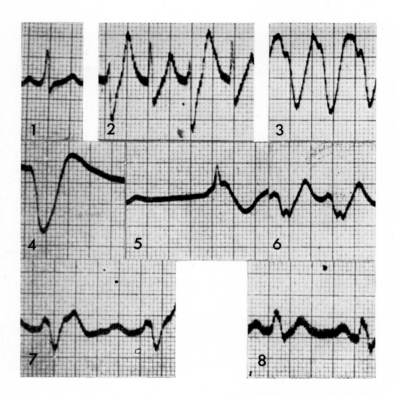

Fig. 91. A case of cardiac arrest occurring during anaesthesia and surgery. Lead II taken in all tracings. 1. Normal ECG 2. Multifocal ventricular extrasystoles 3. ventricular fibrillation 4. Massage contraction 5. Complex initiated by the heart 6. intraventricular conduction defect 7. conduction defect less marked 8. ECG at the end of the operation.

Drugs used to treat an abnormal rhythm should be administered not only under ECG control but under the advice and guidance of a cardiologist. The treatment of fast arrhythmias necessitates the use of such drugs as digitalis, quinidine, procaine amide and lignocaine, while neostigmine is occasionally required. When arrhythmias are slow, as in various forms of heart block, ephedrine, adrenaline, isoprenaline and atropine may be employed. Electrolyte imbalance may play an important part in maintaining an arrhythmia in which case such drugs as potassium chloride, sodium lactate or sodium bicarbonate may help in its control (Smith 1960).

Atrial, nodal, and ventricular extrasystoles which are initiated during a cardiotomy may persist for a day or two into the post-operative period.

The ECG should be checked twenty-four hours post-operatively for evidence of infarction in patients over 50 years of age with known coronary heart disease, hypertension, diabetes mellitus, peripheral vascular disease or abnormal pre-operative ECGs (Driscoll et al 1960).

THE RESPIRATORY UNIT AND THE OXYGEN PRESSURE CHAMBER

The ECG may also be of value in these locations, particularly in patients with severe tetanus, where conduction defects may indicate the onset of myocarditis or inadequate pulmonary ventilation. (Smythe & Bull 1959; Alhady et al 1960; Smythe 1963); and in patients with carbon monoxide poisoning where the ECG picture has been shown to improve rapidly when these patients are given oxygen at a pressure of two atmospheres (Sharp et al 1962).

LIMITATIONS OF THE ECG

The ECG only portrays the electrical activity of the heart and provides no indication of the strength of myocardial contraction and no record of haemodynamic events. Indeed, it has on occasion been known to provide a relatively normal tracing, certainly in a single standard lead, when the heart has ceased to beat effectively as a pump. An illustration of this is shown in Fig. 92. The patient had been clinically dead for some minutes when the relatively normal tracing was recorded and it was not until the lapse of a further half minute that this tracing changed into one of ventricular fibrillation.

On the other hand, the ECG may, on occasion, show grossly bizarre patterns in the presence of an adequate blood pressure. This does not call for panic, but the anaesthetist should ascertain the cause of the abnormal pattern and if possible remove it.

Finally, it should be stressed that the ECG should be used only as an ancillary aid and the anaesthetist should realize that it is no substitute for keen and constant clinical observation before, during

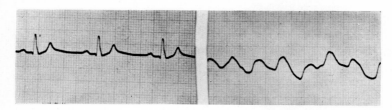

FIG. 92. *Tracings on the left:* Normal ECG tracing but patient clinically dead.

Tracings on the right: Taken 30 seconds later — ventricular fibrillation.

(Lead II)

and after surgery. The colour, BP, pulse rate, capillary refill time and pupil size should be frequently checked and take priority over any ECG tracings, except during periods of elective cardiac arrest.

ARRHYTHMIAS OCCURRING DURING ANAESTHESIA

Type	Causes	Treatment
Extrasystoles		
(a) Atrial	Anoxia	Remove offending
(b) Nodal	CO_2 retention	stimulus
(c) Ventricular	Anaesthetic agents	Ensure adequate oxygen-
	especially chloroform	ation and CO_2 elimina-
	in the presence of	tion
	adrenaline	Correct electrolyte
	Atropine	imbalance and
	Digitalis	metabolic acidosis
	Metabolic derangement	Raise BP and tempera-
	Hypothermia	ture if indicated
	Intubation	Drugs: procaine amide
	Cardiac catheterization	quinidine
	Coronary angiography	lignocaine
	Cardiac surgery	Terminate surgery
Tachycardia		
(a) Supraventricular	Anoxia	Remove offending
(b) Ventricular	Haemorrhage	stimulus
	Drugs: adrenaline	Restore depleted blood
	chlorpromazine	volume
	gallamine	Carotid sinus and eyeball
	atropine	pressure
	Catheter in the heart	Drugs: vasopressors
	Surgical manipulation	digitalis (if not due to
	of the heart	digitalis toxicity)
		procaine amide
		quinidine
		lignocaine
		Terminate surgery

Bradycardia	Irritant anaesthetic vapours	Remove offending stimulus
	Drugs: neostigmine suxamethonium digitalis vasopressors C_3H_6, $ChCl_3$ and halothane	IV atropine
	Overdistension of the lungs in controlled respiration	
	Surgical stimulation of the vagus	
	Traction on extrinsic muscles of eye	
AV Block	Cardiac surgery e.g. mitral valvotomy Repair of VSD Beck operation	Remove offending stimulus e.g. suture involving the bundle of His finger or valvulotome in the heart clamp including a coronary artery
		Insert external or internal pacemaker if AV block is complete and will not respond to drugs such as atropine and isoprenaline
Ventricular Fibrillation	Anoxia Infarction Hypothermia Elective cardiac arrest	Adequate oxygenation and CO_2 elimination
		Cardiac massage
		Restore myocardial tone with adrenaline or $CaCl_2$ and give molar sodium lactate (Dripps *et al* 1961)
		Isoprenaline for 'slow' fibrillation
		Raise temperature, if low
		Electrically defibrillate. If this fails try biochemical defibrillation (Beveridge & Rollason 1963)

REFERENCES

ABRAMS L D., HUDSON W. A. & LIGHTWOOD R. (1960) A surgical approach to the management of heart-block using an inductive coupled artificial cardiac pacemaker. *Lancet*, **i**, 1372

ALHADY S. M. A., BOWLER D. P., REID H. A. & SCOTT L. T. (1960) Total paralysis regime in severe tetanus. *Brit. med. J.* **i**, 540

ALLAN C. M., CULLEN W. G. & GILLIES D. M. M. (1961) Ventricular fibrillation in a burned boy. *Canadian M.A.J.* **85**, 432

ALTSCHULE M. D. & SULZBACH W. M. (1947) Tolerance of the human heart to acidosis: reversible changes in RS-T interval during severe acidosis caused by administration of carbon dioxide. *Amer. Heart J.* **33**, 458

ANTONIUS R. A., NEWMAN W., CRECCA A. D. & MASSARELLI L. D. (1956) The selection of cases of coronary heart disease suitable for surgical treatment. *Dis. Chest.* **29**, 305

ARCURI R. A., NEWMAN W. & BURSTEIN C. L. (1953) Electrocardiographic studies during endotracheal intubation. V: Effects during general anesthesia and hexylcaine hydrochloride topical spray. *Anesthesiology*, **14**, 46

ASCHNER B. (1908) Über einen bisher noch nicht beschriebenen Reflex vom Auge auf Kreislauf und Atmung. *Wien. klin. Wschr.* **21**, 1529

ASERMAN D. (1953) Controlled hypotension in neurosurgery. *Brit. med. J.* **1**, 961

ASHMAN R. (1948) The physiological and physical aspects of the electrocardiogram. In *The Chest and Heart*, ed. Myers J. A. & McKinley C. N. Vol. II, p. 1421. Charles C. Thomas, Springfield, Illinois.

AVERILL K. H. & LAMB L. E. (1959) Less commonly recognised actions of atropine on cardiac rhythm. *Amer. J. med. Sci.* **237**, 304

BARRETO R. S. (1960) Effect of intravenously administered succinylcholine upon cardiac rate and rhythm. *Anesthesiology*, **21**, 401

BAYLEY R. H. (1943) On certain applications of modern electrocardiographic theory to the interpretation of electrocardiograms which indicate myocardial disease. *Amer. Heart J.* **26**, 769

BECKMAN M. & HALLDIN M. (1960) The effect of succinylcholine on cardiac rhythm. Preliminary report. *Opusc. med. (Stockh.)* **5**, 322

BELLET S., HAMDEN G., SOMLYO A. & LARA R. (1959) A reversal of the cardio-toxic effects of procaine amide by molar sodium lactate. *Amer. J. med. Sci.* **237,** 177

BENAZON D. (1960) The experimental and clinical use of profound hypothermia. *Anaesthesia,* **15,** 134

BENAZON D. (1962) Pressor drugs. An appraisal of their place in anaesthetic practice. *Anaesthesia,* **17,** 344

BEVERIDGE M.E. & ROLLASON W.N. (1963) Biochemical Defibrillation. *Lancet,* ii, 1281.

BLACK G.W., LINDE H.W., DRIPPS R.D. & PRICE H.L. (1959) Circulatory changes accompanying respiratory acidosis during halothane anaesthesia in man. *Brit. J. Anaesth.* **31,** 238

BOSOMWORTH P.P., ZIEGLER C.H. & JACOBY J. (1958) The oculo-cardiac reflex in eye muscle surgery. *Anesthesiology,* **19,** 7

BOYAN C.P. & HOWLAND W.S. (1961) Blood temperature: A critical factor in massive transfusion. *Anesthesiology,* **22,** 559

BOYAN C.P. & HOWLAND W.S. (1962) Problems related to massive blood replacement. *Curr. Res. Anesth.* **41,** 497

BRINDLE G.F., GILBERT R.G.B. & MILLER R.A. (1957) Use of fluothane in anaesthesia for neurosurgery; preliminary report. *Canad. Anaesth. Soc. J.* **4,** 265

BUCKLEY J.J. & JACKSON J.A. (1961) Post-operative cardiac arrythmias. *Anesthesiology,* **22,** 723

BUNKER J.P., BENDIXEN H.H. & MURPHY A.J. (1962) The haemodynamic effects of intravenously administered sodium citrate. *New Engl. J. Med.* **266,** 372

BURNAP T.K., GALLA S.J. & VANDAM L.D. (1958) Anesthetic, circulatory and respiratory effects of fluothane. *Anesthesiology,* **19,** 307

BURSTEIN C.L. LOPINTO F.J. & NEWMAN W. (1950a) Electrocardiographic studies during endotracheal intubation. I: Effects during usual routine technics. *Anesthesiology,* **11,** 224

BURSTEIN C.L., WOLOSHIN G. & NEWMAN W. (1950b) Electrocardiographic studies during endotracheal intubation. II: Effects during general anesthesia and intravenous procaine. *Anesthesiology,* **11,** 299

BURSTEIN C.L., ZAINO G. & NEWMAN W. (1951) Electrocardiographic studies during endotracheal intubation. III: Effects during general anesthesia and intravenous diethylaminoethanol. *Anesthesiology,* **12,** 411

BUSH G.H., GRAHAM H.A.P., LITTLEWOOD A.H.M. & SCOTT L.B. (1962) Danger of suxamethonium and endotracheal intubation in anaesthesia for burns. *Brit. med. J.* ii, 1081

CAMERINI F., GUGLIELMI F. & PIZZOLI R. (1952) Studio elettrocardiografico nel corso di interventi operatori in ipotensione controllata. *G. ital. Anest.* **18,** 505

CAMERINI F., MARTINALI E. & MORENA L. (1958) Elektrokardiographische Untersuchungen Während Künstlicher Hypotonic mit Trimetaphan. *Anaesthesist*, **7**, 327

CANNARD T.H., DRIPPS R.D., HELWIG J. JR. & ZINSSER H.F. (1960) The electrocardiogram during anesthesia and surgery. *Anesthesiology*, **21**, 194

CLARKE N.E. (1941) The action of calcium on the human electrocardiogram. *Amer. Heart J.* **22**, 367

CLEMENT A.J. (1962) Atropine premedication for electric convulsion therapy. *Brit. med. J.* **i**, 228

CONVERSE J.G., LANDMESSER C.M. & HARMEL M.H. (1952) Electrocardiographic changes during extubation. A study of electrocardiographic patterns during endotracheal anesthesia including those seen during intubation, endotracheal suction, and particularly extubation. *Anesthesiology*, **13**, 163

CRAYTHORNE N.W.B., TURNDORF H. & DRIPPS R.D. (1960) Changes in pulse rate and rhythm associated with the use of succinylcholine in anesthetised children. *Anesthesiology*, **21**, 465

CURRIE T.T., CASS N.M. & HICKS J.D. (1962) The scope of surface cooling. An experimental study using quinidine as a prophylactic against ventricular fibrillation. *Anaesthesia*, **17**, 46

CURTISS H.J. & COLE K.S. (1941) Membrane resting and action potentials of the squid giant axon. *Amer. J. Physiol.* **133**, 254

DALE W.A. (1952) Cardiac arrest: review and report of 12 cases. *Ann. Surg.* **135**, 375

DANCE C.L. JR., BOOZER J., NEWMAN W. & BURSTEIN C.L. (1956) Electrocardiographic studies during endotracheal intubation. VII: Evipal sodium induction. *Anesthesiology*, **17**, 730

DAVISON M.H.A. (1951) Discussion on the use of hypotensive drugs in surgery. *Proc. Roy. Soc. Med.* **44**, 832

DAWSON B., THEYE R.A. & KIRKLIN J.W. (1960) Halothane in open cardiac operations; a technique for use with extra corporeal circulation. *Curr. Res. Anesth.* **39**, 59

DEACOCK A.R. DE C. & OXER H.F. (1962) The prevention of reflex tachycardia during ophthalmic surgery. *Brit. J. Anaesth.* **34**, 451

DELANEY E.J. (1958) Cardiac irregularities during induction with halothane. *Brit. J. Anaesth.* **30**, 188

DENSON J.S. & JOSEPH S.I. (1954) Cardiac rhythm and endotracheal intubation — a clarification. *Anesthesiology*, **15**, 650

DOBKIN A.B. (1949) The effects of anticholinergic drugs on the cardiac vagus: I. Clinical observations in patients undergoing electroshock treatment. *Canad. Anaesth. Soc. J.* **6**, 51

DRIPPS R.D., ECKENHOFF J.E. & VAN DAM L.D. (1961) *Introduction to Anesthesia*, 2nd edit., p. 332. Saunders, London

DRISCOLL A.C., HOBIKA J.H., ETSTEN E. & PROGER S. (1960) Myocardial infarction and other E.C.G. changes in the post-operative period. *Bull. Tufts-New Engl. med. Center*, **6**, 1

EBNER H., BARCOHANA J. & BARTOSHUK A.K. (1960) Influence of post-spinal hypotension on the fetal electrocardiogram. *Amer. J. Obstet. Gynec.* **80**, 569

EINTHOVEN W. (1903) Die galvanometrische Registrirung des Menschlichen elektrokardiogramms, Zugleich eine Beurtheilung der Amvendung des Cupillar elektrometers in der Physiologie, *Pflügers Arch. ges. Physiol.* **99**, 472

EMSLIE-SMITH D., SNEDDEN G.E. & STIRLING G.R. (1959) The significance of changes in the electrocardiogram in hypothermia. *Brit. Heart J.* **21**, 343

ENDERBY G.E.H. (1951) Discussion on the use of hypotensive drugs in surgery. *Proc. Roy. Soc. Med.* **44**, 829

FISHER K. & WINSOR T. (1952) Contributions of electrocardiography to anesthesia for chest surgery. *Anesthesiology*, **13**, 147

FOSTER B. (1961) Suxamethonium and cardiac rhythm. *Brit. med. J.* i, 129

GAIN E.A. (1962) The problem of cardiac collapse associated with the massive transfusion of citrated blood. *Canad. Anaesth. Soc. J.* **9**, 207

GARDNER W.J. (1946) The control of bleeding during operations by induced hypotension. *J. Amer. med. Ass.*, **132**, 572.

GAUTHIER J., BOSOMWORTH P., PAGE D., MOORE F., & HAMELBERG W. (1962) Effect of endotracheal intubation on ECG patterns during halothane anesthesia. *Curr. Res. Anesth.* **41**, 466.

GILLESPIE N.A. (1951) The relation of intubation to post-operative respiratory complications. *Anaesthesia*, **6**, 206

GLASS H., SHAW G. & SMITH G. (1963) An implantable cardiac pacemaker allowing rate control. *Lancet*, i, 684

GOODMAN L.S. & GILMAN A. (1955) *The pharmacological basis of therapeutics*. 2nd edn, p. 59. Macmillan, New York

GORDON E. & LADENHEIM J.C. (1955) Controlled hypotension in neurosurgery. Clinical experiences with arfonad and hibernal. *Acta chir. scand.* **109**, 488

GOTTLIEB J.D. & SWEET R.B. (1963) The antagonism of curare: The cardiac effects of atropine and neostigmine. *Canad. Anaesth. Soc. J.* **10**, 114.

HAID B. (1954) Klinik und 'Low Pressure' mit Cesonderer Berücksichtigung von EKG — Veränderungen. *Anaesthestist*, **3**, 49

HEARD J.D. & STRAUSS A.E. (1918) A report on the electrocardiographic study of two cases of nodal rhythm exhibiting R-P intervals. *Amer. J. med. Sci.* **155**, 238

HENDERSON A.G., MACKETT J. & MASHETER H.C. (1958) The effect of thiopentone and buthalitone upon the QT interval in the electrocardiogram. *Brit. J. Anaesth.* **30**, 302

HILL I.G.W. (1932a) Cardiac irregularities during chloroform anaesthesia. *Lancet*, **i**, 1139

HILL I.G.W. (1932b) The human heart in anaesthesia; an electrocardiographic study. *Edinb. med. J.* **39**, 533

HOLLOWAY K.B., HOLMES F. & HIDER C.F. (1961) Guanethidine in hypotensive anaesthesia: Clinical study on patients undergoing microsurgery of the middle ear. *Brit. J. Anaesth.* **33**, 648

HORTON J.A.G. (1955) Electrocardiographic findings during laryngoscopy and endotracheal intubation. *Brit. J. Anaesth.* **27**, 326

HOWAT D.D.C. (1963) Anaesthesia for the insertion of indwelling artificial pacemakers. *Lancet*, **i**, 855

HOWLAND W.S., JACOBS R.G. & GAULET A.H. (1960) An evaluation of calcium administration during rapid blood replacement. *Curr. Res. Anesth.* **39**, 557

JACOBSON E. & ADELMAN M.H. (1954) The electrocardiographic effects of intravenous administration of neostigmine and atropine during cyclopropane anesthesia. *Anesthesiology*, **15**, 407

JACOBY J., ZEIGLER C., HAMELBERG W., MOGG A., KLASSEN K. & FLORY F. (1955) Cardiac arrhythmia; effect of vagal stimulation and hypoxia. *Anesthesiology*, **16**, 1004

JAMES A., COULTER R.L. & SAUNDERS J.W. (1953) Controlled hypotension in neurosurgery. *Lancet*, **i**, 414

JONES R.E., DEUTSCH S. & TURNDORF H. (1961) Effects of atropine on cardiac rhythm in conscious and anesthetised man. *Anesthesiology*, **22**, 67

JOHNSTONE M. (1950) Cyclopropane anaesthesia and ventricular arrhythmias. *Brit. Heart J.* **12**, 239

JOHNSTONE M. (1951) Pethidine and general anaesthesia. *Brit. med. J.* **ii**, 943

JOHNSTONE M. (1953) Adrenaline and noradrenaline during anaesthesia. *Anaesthesia*, **8**, 32

JOHNSTONE M. (1955) Relaxants and the human cardiovascular system. *Anaesthesia*, **10**, 122

JOHNSTONE M. (1956) Electrocardiography during anaesthesia. *Brit. J. Anaesth.* **28**, 579

JOHNSTONE M. & NISBET H.I.A. (1961) Ventricular arrhythmia during halothane anaesthesia. *Brit. J. Anaesth.* **33**, 9

KENDALL B., FARRELL D.M. & KANE H.A. (1962) Fetal radioelectrocardiography: a new method of fetal electrocardiography. *Amer. J. Obstet. Gynec.* **83**, 1629

KERWIN A.J., MCLEAN R. & TAGELAAR H. (1960) A method for the accurate placement of chest electrodes in the taking of serial electrocardiographic tracings. *Canad. med. Ass. J.* **82**, 258

KÖLLIKER A. & MÜLLER H. (1856) Nachweis der negativen Schwantung des Muskelstroms am Naturlich sich contrahirenden Muskel. *Verh. phys.-med. Ges. Wurzb.* **6**, 528

KING B.D., HARRIS L.C. JR., GREIFENSTEIN F.E., ELDER J.D. JR. & DRIPPS R.D. (1951) Reflex circulatory responses to direct laryngoscopy and tracheal intubation performed during general anesthesia. *Anesthesiology*, 12, 556

KIRSCH R.E., SAMET P., KUGEL V. & AXELROD S. (1957) Electrocardiographic changes during ocular surgery and their prevention by retrobulbar injection. *A.M.A. Arch. Ophth.* 58, 348

KRUMBHAAR E.B. (1918) Electrocardiographic observations in toxic goiter. *Amer. J. med. Sci.* 155, 175

KURTZ C.M., BENNETT J.H. & SHAPIRO H.H. (1936) Electrocardiographic studies during surgical anesthesia. *J. Amer. med. Ass.* 106, 434

LARKS S.D. (1961) *Fetal Electrocardiography.* 1st edn. Charles C.Thomas, Springfield, Illinois

LEATHAM A.G., CORK P. & DAVIES J.G. (1956) External electric stimulator for treatment of ventricular standstill. *Lancet*, ii, 1185

LEIGH M.D., McCOY D.D., BELTON M.K. & LEWIS G.B. (1957) Bradycardia following intravenous administration of succinylcholine chloride to infants and children. *Anesthesiology*, 18, 698

LE VEEN H.H., PASTERNACK H.S., LUSTRIN I., SHAPIRO R.B., BECKER E. & HELFT A.H. (1960) Hemorrhage and transfusion as the major cause of cardiac arrest. *J. Amer. med. Ass.* 173, 770

LEVY A.G. (1913) The exciting causes of ventricular fibrillation in animals under chloroform anaesthesia. *Heart*, 4, 319

LEVY A.G. (1914) The genesis of ventricular extrasystoles, under chloroform with special reference to consecutive ventricular fibrillation. *Heart*, 5, 299

LUDBROOK J. & WYNN, V. (1958) Citrate intoxication. A clinical and experimental study. *Brit. med. J.* ii, 523

LUPPRIAN K.G. & CHURCHILL-DAVIDSON H.C. (1960) Effect of suxamethonium on cardiac rhythm. *Brit. med. J.* ii, 1774

LURIE A.A., JONES R.E., LINDE H.W., PRICE M.L., DRIPPS R.D. & PRICE H.L. (1958) Cyclopropane anesthesia; cardiac rate and rhythm during steady levels of cyclopropane anesthesia in man at normal and elevated end-expiratory CO_2 tensions. *Anesthesiology*, 19, 457

LYNN R.B., SANCETTA S.M., SIMEONE F.A. & SCOTT R.W. (1952) Observations on the circulation in high spinal anesthesia. *Surgery*, 32, 195

MALLINSON F.B. & COOMBS S.K. (1960) A hazard of anaesthesia in ophthalmic surgery. *Lancet*, i, 574

MALSTRÖM G., NORDENSTRÖM B., NORLANDER O. & SENNING A. (1960) The coronary patient as an anaesthetic risk. Results of anaesthetic procedures for coronary angiography with a technique including periods of hypotension. *Acta anaesth. scand. Suppl. VI*, p. 24

MANDOW G.A., ARDEN G.P. & STONEHAM F.J.R. (1954) Hypotension induced with hexamethonium bromide during anaesthesia. *Brit. J. Anaesth.* 26, 26

MARSHALL M. (1962) Potassium intoxication from blood and plasma transfusions. *Anaesthesia*, **17**, 145

MARTIN K.H. (1958) Die Wirkung Des Succinylcholine auf den Herzohythmus. *Atti XI Congr. Soc. ital. Anest.*, p. 362

MASON A.A. & PELMORE J.F. (1953) Combined use of hexamethonium, bromide and procaine amide in controlled hypotension. *Brit. med. J.* **i**, 250

MAZZIA V.D.B., BRONSON S.R. & ARTUSIO J.F. JR. (1956) The use of thiophanium derivative for controlled hypotension in intracranial operations. *Ann. Surg.* **143**, 81

MCARDLE L. (1959) Electrocardiographic studies during the inhalation of 30% CO_2 in man. *Brit. J. Anaesth.* **31**, 142

MENDELSOHN D., MACDONALD D.W., NOGUEIRA C. & KAY E.B. (1960) Anesthesia for open heart surgery. *Curr. Res. Anesth.* **39**, 110

MILLAR R.A., GILBERT R.G.B. & BRINDLE G.F. (1958) Ventricular tachycardia during halothane anaesthesia. *Anaesthesia*, **13**, 164

MILSTEIN B.B. (1961) Cardiac resuscitation. *Brit. J. Anaesth.* **33**, 498

MORTON H.J.V. & THOMAS E.T. (1958) Effect of atropine on the heart rate. *Lancet*, **ii**, 1313

MURTAGH G.P. (1960) Controlled hypotension with halothane. *Anaesthesia*, **15**, 235

NOBLE M.J. & DERRICK W.S. (1959) Changes in the electrocardiogram during induction of anaesthesia and endotracheal intubation. *Canad. Anaes. Soc. J.* **6**, 267

NOORDIJK J.A., OEY F.T.I. & TEBRA W. (1961) Myocardial electrodes and the danger of ventricular fibrillation. *Lancet*, **i**, 975

NOSWORTHY M.D. (1938) Some respiratory disturbances during general anaesthesia. *Anaesthesia*, **3**, 86

ORTH O.S. (1958) In *Pharmacology in Medicine*. 2nd edn. Chapters 5 & 6. Ed. V.A.Drill. McGraw-Hill, New York

ORTON R.H. & MORRIS K.N. (1959) Deliberate circulatory arrest: The use of halothane and heparin for direct vision intracardiac surgery. *Thorax*, **14**, 39

OSBORN J.J. (1953) Experimental hypothermia; respiratory and blood pH changes in relation to cardiac function. *Amer. J. Physiol.* **175**, 389

PAYNE J.P. & PLANTEVIN O.M. (1962) Action du fluothane sur le coeur. *Anesth. Analg.* **19**, 45

PETERS N.S., NEWMAN W. & BURSTEIN C.L. (1951) Electrocardiographic studies during endotracheal intubation. IV: Effects during cyclopropane or cyclopropane-ether anesthesia and intravenous procaine amide. *Anesthesiology*, **12**, 673

PHILLIPS H.S. (1954) Physiologic changes noted with the use of succinylcholine chloride, as a muscle relaxant during endotracheal intubation. *Curr. Res. Anesth.* **33**, 165

POOLER H.E. (1957) Atropine, neostigmine and sudden deaths. *Anaesthesia*, **12**, 198

PORTAL R.W., DAVIES J.G., LEATHAM A.G. & SIDDONS A.H.M. (1962) Artificial pacing for heart block. *Lancet*, **ii**, 1369

PORTAL R.W., DAVIES J.G., ROBINSON B.F. & LEATHAM A.G. (1963) Notes on cardiac resuscitation including external cardiac massage. *Brit. med. J.* **i**, 636

PRICE H.L., LURIE A.A., JONES R.E., PRICE M.L. & LINDE H.W. (1958) Cyclopropane anesthesia: epinephrine and norepinephrine in initiation of ventricular arrythmias by carbon dioxide inhalation. *Anesthesiology*, **19**, 619

PRINZMETAL M., CORDAY E., BRILL I.S., SELLERS A.L., OBLATH R.W., FLIEG W.A. & KRUGH H.E. (1950) Mechanics of the auricular arrhythmias. *Circulation*, **1**, 241

REID L.C. & BRACE D.E. (1940) Irritation of the respiratory tract and its reflex effect upon the heart. *Surg. Gynec. Obstet.* **70**, 157

RIDING J.E. & ROBINSON J.S. (1961) The safety of neostigmine. *Anaesthesia*, **16**, 346

ROBSON J.G. & SHERIDAN C.A. (1957) Preliminary investigations with fluothane. *Curr. Res. Anesth.* **36**, 62

ROLLASON W.N. (1953) Anesthesia and the 'bloodless' field. *Curr. Res. Anesth.* **32**, 294

ROLLASON W.N. (1957) Atropine, neostigmine and sudden deaths. *Anaesthesia*, **12**, 364

ROLLASON W.N. (1958) Side effects of antidote drugs. *Atti XI Congr. Soc. ital. Anes.*, p. 546

ROLLASON W.N. (1960) Halothane and hypotension. *Anaesthesia*, **15**, 199

ROLLASON W.N. (1963) Halothane and phaeochromocytoma (in press).

ROLLASON W.N. & CUMMING A.R.R. (1956) The electrocardiogram in hypotensive anaesthesia. *Anaesthesia*, **11**, 319

ROLLASON W.N., DUNDAS C.R. & MILNE R.G. (1963) ECG & EEG changes during hypotensive anaesthesia for 'no catheter' prostatectomy (in press).

ROLLASON W.N. & HOUGH J.M. (1957a) A possible fallacy in single lead electrocardiography. *Lancet*, **ii**, 245

ROLLASON W.N. & HOUGH J.M. (1957b) Electrocardiographic studies during endotracheal intubation and inflation of the cuff. *Brit. J. Anaesth.* **29**, 363

ROLLASON W.N. & HOUGH J.M. (1958) Thiopentone induction and the electrocardiogram. *Brit. J. Aneasth.* **30**, 50

ROLLASON, W.N. & HOUGH J.M. (1959) Some electrocardiographic studies during hypotensive anaesthesia. *Brit. J. Anaesth.* **31**, 66

ROLLASON W.N. & HOUGH J.M. (1960a) The influence of chlorpromazine and hydergine on pethidine and scopolamine premedication. *Brit. J. Anaesth.* **33**, 580

ROLLASON W.N. & HOUGH J.M. (1960b) A study of hypotensive anaesthesia in the elderly. *Brit. J. Anaesth.* **32**, 276

ROLLASON W. N. & HOUGH J. M. (1960c) Is it safe to employ hypotensive anaesthesia in the elderly? *Brit. J. Anaesth.* **32,** 286

ROLLASON W. N. & LATHAM J. W. (1963) Anaesthesia for Intracranial aneurysms. *Anaesthesia,* **18,** 498

ROLLASON W. N. & PARKES J. (1957) Anaesthesia, hyperventilation and the peripheral blood. *Anaesthesia,* **12,** 61

ROSE G. A. (1961) A calliper for siting the precordial leads in electrocardiography. *Lancet,* **i,** 31

ROSEN M. & ROE R. B. (1963) Adrenaline infiltration during halothane anaesthesia. *Brit. J. Anaesth.* **35,** 51

ROSNER S., NEWMAN W. & BURSTEIN C. L. (1953) Electrocardiographic studies during endotracheal intubation. VI: Effects during anesthesia with thiopental sodium combined with a muscle relaxant. *Anesthesiology,* **14,** 591

ROSS E. B. T. (1962) General anaesthesia in complete heart block. *Brit. J. Anaesth.* **34,** 102

RUMBALL C. A. (1963) An Axis-Deviation Calculator. *Lancet,* **2,** 20

SAGARMINAGA J. & WYNANDS J. E. (1963) Atropine and the electrical activity of the heart during induction of anaesthesia in children. *Canad. Anaes. Soc. J.* **10,** 328

SCHAMROTH L. (1961) *An Introduction to Electrocardiography,* p. 11. Blackwell Scientific Publications, Oxford

SCOTT, J. C. & BALOURDAS T. A. (1959) An analysis of coronary flow and related factors following vagotomy atropine and sympathectomy. *Circul. Res.* **7,** 162

SCURR C. F. (1950) Reflex circulatory disturbances during anaesthesia. *Anaesthesia,* **5,** 67

SHARP G. R., LEDINGHAM I. McA. & NORMAN J. N. (1962) The application of oxygen at 2 atmospheres pressure in the treatment of acute anoxia. *Anaesthesia,* **17,** 136

SHEPHERD R. J. (1961) The design of a cardiac defibrillator. *Brit. Heart J.* **23,** 7

SMITH K. S. (1960) Cardiac arrythmias. *Brit. med J.* **i,** 638

SMITH R. S. & NOLAN F. W. (1950) Cardiac arrest incident to surgical anesthesia. *Northw. Med., Seattle,* **49,** 682

SMYTH C. N. (1962) Foetal response to adrenaline and noradrenaline. *Brit. med. J.* **i,** 940

SMYTHE P. M. & BULL A. (1959) The treatment of tetanus neonatorum with intermittent positive pressure respiration. *Brit. med. J.* **ii,** 107

SMYTHE P. M. (1963) Studies on neonatal tetanus and in pulmonary compliance of the totally relaxed infant. *Brit. med. J.* **i,** 565

SORENSON E. J. & GILMORE J. E. (1956) Cardiac arrest during strabismus surgery. *Amer. J. Ophthal.* **41,** 748

STEPHEN C. R., MARTIN R. & NOWILL W. K. (1953) Cardiovascular reactions to surital, pentothal or evipal combined with muscle relaxants for rapid anesthesia induction. *Curr. Res. Anesth.* **32,** 361

STIRLING J.B. (1955) Anaesthesia with hypotension for fenestration. *Brit. J. Anaesth.* **27,** 80

SWERDLOW M. & WADE H.J. (1953) The effects of hexamethonium iodide in the electrocardiograph in anaesthetized subjects. *Brit. J. Anaesth.* **27,** 80

SZABO G., SOLTI F., REV J., REFI Z. & MEGYESI K. (1957) Die Wirkung von Chlorpromazin auf die Hypoxie des Herzmuskels. *Z. Kreisl.-Forsch.* **46,** 197

VAN BERGEN F.H., BUCKLEY J.J., FRENCH L.A., DOBKIN A.B. & BROWN I.A. (1954) Physiologic alterations associated with hexamethonium induced hypotension. *Anesthesiology,* **15,** 5

WALLER A.D. (1887) A demonstration on man of electromotive changes accompanying the heart's beat. *J. Physiol.* **8,** 229

WATERS R.M. & GILLESPIE N.A. (1944) Deaths in the operating room. *Anesthesiology,* **5,** 113

WEISS W.A. (1960) Intravenous use of lidocaine for ventricular arrythmias. *Curr. Res. Anesth.* **39,** 369

WEISS W.A. & BAILEY C.P. (1960) Extracorporeal circulation in cardiac surgery. *Curr. Res. Anesth.* **39,** 438

WENGER VON R., DONEFF D. & VYSLONZIE E. (1953) Zur Kreislaufwirkung ganglien blockierender Stoffe. *Dtsch. med. Wschr.* **78,** 322

WYMAN J.B. (1953) The use of pentamethonium and hexamethonium salts in major surgery. *Hunterian Lecture, Royal College of Surgeons of England, March 12th*

INDEX